Ian C. Scott • James B. Galloway
David L. Scott

Inflammatory Arthritis in Clinical Practice

Second Edition

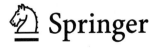

 Springer

Ian C. Scott
Molecular and Cellular Biology
of Inflammation
King's College London
London
UK

James B. Galloway
Rheumatology
King's College Hospital
London
UK

David L. Scott
Rheumatology
King's College Hospital
London
UK

ISBN 978-1-4471-6647-4   ISBN 978-1-4471-6648-1   (eBook)
DOI 10.1007/978-1-4471-6648-1
Springer London Heidelberg New York Dordrecht

Library of Congress Control Number: 2015932095

Printed on acid-free paper

Springer is part of Springer Science+Business Media (www.springer.com)

Preface

The inflammatory arthropathies are a group of conditions characterised by pain and swelling of the joints. The commonest types comprise rheumatoid arthritis (RA), psoriatic arthritis (PsA), ankylosing spondylitis (AS) and reactive arthritis. In most instances they represent long-term conditions, which require treatment with immunosuppressive drugs. Unless adequately managed they can have major impacts on patients resulting in pain, disability and an impaired quality of life.

Over the last three decades the assessment and diagnosis of inflammatory arthritis has rapidly and radically changed. This has accelerated in the last few years with a series of major developments. These span new diagnostic tests such as antibodies to citrullinated protein antigens (ACPA) in RA, novel imaging approaches such as the high-resolution ultrasound power Doppler modality, and new treatments, particularly biologics.

There has also been a major shift in the manner in which inflammatory arthritis is viewed and treated. The historical Spa hospital ethos of bed rest and hydrotherapy has been completely cast aside in favour of early intensive treatment with combination disease-modifying anti-rheumatic drugs (DMARDs) and biologics. The end result has been improved patient outcomes.

There are still many challenges to overcome in the management of inflammatory arthritis patients. Firstly, as early treatment results in better outcomes, an improved ability to diagnose and treat these diseases at an early stage is needed. Secondly, as patients have a variable disease course, biomarkers are required that predict an individual's likely disease severity; such markers could guide decisions on treatment intensity. Thirdly, different patients respond to different drugs; methods are therefore needed that can predict what medications someone is likely to benefit from, providing tailored treatment. Finally, as current tools to measure disease activity and severity in routine clinics have limitations, such as the "floor-effect" of joint counts, improved methods to measure the impact of inflammatory arthritis are required.

Understanding the key components of the diagnosis, assessment and management of inflammatory arthritis patients is essential to improving patient care. This book aims to cover these areas. It places inflammatory arthritis into a historical context; deals with the epidemiology, pathology, clinical assessment and investigation of inflammatory arthritis patients; and provides a comprehensive overview of currently available treatment options. It provides insight into stratified medicine, an area of emerging importance in the management of heterogeneous diseases like RA. Finally, it provides an overview of what treatment strategies are in development.

London, UK   Ian C. Scott
London, UK   James B. Galloway
London, UK   David L. Scott

Contents

Abbreviations

ACPA	Antibodies to citrullinated protein antigens
ACR	American College of Rheumatology
ANA	Anti-nuclear antibody
AS	Ankylosing spondylitis
ASAS	Assessment of Spondyloarthritis International Society
BASDAI	Bath Ankylosing Spondylitis Disease Activity Index
BASFI	Bath Ankylosing Spondylitis Functional Index
BTK	Bruton's tyrosine kinase
CARDERA	Combination Anti-Rheumatic Drugs in Early RA
CASPAR	Classification Criteria for Psoriatic Arthritis
CDAI	Clinical Disease Activity Index
COX	Cyclo-oxygenase
CRP	C-reactive protein
CT	Computerised tomography
DAS	Disease activity score
DEXA	Dual-energy X-ray absorptiometry
DIP	Distal interphalangeal
DMARD	Disease-modifying anti-rheumatic drug
dsDNA	Double stranded DNA
ELISA	Enzyme-linked immunosorbent assays
ESR	Erythrocyte sedimentation rate
EULAR	European League Against Rheumatism
HAQ	Health Assessment Questionnaire
IBD	Inflammatory bowel disease
IgG	Immunoglobulin G

ILD	Interstitial lung disease
JAK	Janus kinase
MBDA	Multi-biomarker disease activity
MRI	Magnetic resonance imaging
NICE	National Institute for Health and Care Excellence
NSAID	Non-steroidal anti-inflammatory drug
OA	Osteoarthritis
PDE4	Phosphodiesterase 4
PsARC	Psoriatic Arthritis Response Criteria
RA	Rheumatoid arthritis
RF	Rheumatoid factor
RRP	Rapid radiological progression
SDAI	Simplified Disease Activity Index
SE	Shared epitope
SLE	Systemic lupus erythematosus
SMR	Standardised mortality ratio
STAT	Signal Transducer and Activator of Transcription
SyK	Spleen tyrosine kinase
TENS	Transcutaneous electrical nerve stimulation
TNF-α	Tumour necrosis factor-alpha
VAS	Visual analogue scale

Chapter 1
An Overview of Inflammatory Arthritis

Abstract Inflammatory arthritis spans a number of diseases. The most prevalent is rheumatoid arthritis (RA). Others include psoriatic arthritis (PsA), reactive arthritis, ankylosing spondylitis (AS) and arthritis in patients with inflammatory bowel disease (IBD). All represent complex disorders, arising from genetic and environmental risk factors. Their treatment is broadly similar, which is the primary reason for considering them together under the umbrella term of "inflammatory arthropathies". There is no single diagnostic test for any of the inflammatory arthropathies. Classification criteria exist, which provide a standardised approach for identifying individuals with a high probability of having a disease for enrolment into research studies. They are often used in clinical practice to aid diagnosis although the gold standard remains the opinion of an experienced rheumatologist. This chapter will provide an overview of the different types of inflammatory arthritis, their historical perspectives, and how they are diagnosed and classified.

Keywords Inflammatory Arthritis • Historical Perspective • Diagnosis • Classification Criteria

I.C. Scott et al., *Inflammatory Arthritis in Clinical Practice*,
DOI 10.1007/978-1-4471-6648-1_1,
© Springer-Verlag London 2015

Introduction

The inflammatory arthropathies are a group of disorders characterised by joint pain and swelling. Their similar treatments, which include disease-modifying anti-rheumatic drugs (DMARDs) and biologic agents, mean they are often considered together. Their serological and extra-articular manifestations help to differentiate them. This chapter will provide an overview of the inflammatory arthropathies, with a specific focus on their subtypes and how they are diagnosed.

What Are the Inflammatory Arthropathies?

Inflammatory arthritis spans a number of diseases. The most prevalent is rheumatoid arthritis (RA). Others include psoriatic arthritis (PsA), reactive arthritis, ankylosing spondylitis (AS) and arthritis in patients with inflammatory bowel disease (IBD).

A number of disorders in which inflammatory arthritis is sometimes seen, are not usually considered to be a part of the inflammatory arthropathies. These disorders include:

- Arthritis occurring in patients with connective tissue diseases such as systemic lupus erythematosus (SLE) and scleroderma.
- Arthritis due to crystals, mainly gout and pyrophosphate deposition disease.
- Osteoarthritis (OA), which although usually non-inflammatory, can sometimes have inflammatory features.
- Arthritis due to known viral infections
- Bacterial arthritis and arthritis due to other infective agents.
- A number of uncommon disorders, like adult onset Still's disease.

The known causal factors for inflammatory arthritis include genetic risks (particularly in RA and AS), exposure to infection (particularly in reactive arthritis), environmental factors (particularly smoking in RA) and demographic factors (such as age and sex). Most of the diseases are thought to involve autoimmune triggers and immunological mechanisms. There has been extensive speculation about the roles of infective or viral triggers, but no firm conclusions have been reached.

Treatment of these disorders is broadly similar. All respond to symptomatic treatment with analgesics and anti-inflammatory drugs. DMARDs and biologics are often used to both improve symptoms and reduce arthritis disease activity. Non-pharmacological therapies such as exercise and physiotherapy are also recommended. The similar management of these diseases is the main reason for considering them together under the umbrella term of "inflammatory arthropathies".

The spondyloarthropathies are best considered to form a spectrum of diseases characterised by several key features comprising enthesitis, iritis, spinal involvement, the presence of *HLA-B27* and absence of rheumatoid factor (RF). Overlap between these disorders is common with many AS patients having microscopic colitis on colonic biopsy. To an extent it is the presence of associated features outside the joints (termed extra-articular features) that differentiates them. However, in many patients it may be difficult to tell them apart, and often they are considered to be undifferentiated.

Historical Perspectives

Most types of inflammatory arthritis were identified in the nineteenth century, though their exact classification was only finalised in the last 50 years. Prior to 1850 there was considerable uncertainty about how to differentiate different forms of arthritis, and a number of complex, somewhat confusing names were used, such as chronic rheumatic gout. Rheumatic fever, which was commonplace at that time, also caused considerable uncertainly.

The concept of "rheumatoid arthritis" dates from Victorian times and the term was introduced by Sir Archibald Garrod, an academic clinician in London, to distinguish the disease from gout and rheumatic fever. It took many years before the term RA achieved universal recognition. It was not officially taken up by the Empire Rheumatism Council until the 1920s and by the American Rheumatism Association in the 1940s.

The roots of seronegative arthritis can be traced back further to antiquity. AS was present in ancient Egypt and has been identified in mummified remains. There is evidence that several pharaohs including Rameses II ("The Great", 1290–1221BC) had AS. PsA may also have been an ancient disease; skeletons from early Christian society, in a fifth century AD Byzantine monastery in the Judean Desert contained features of PsA. Reactive arthritis has a more recent provenance. Although there have been suggestions that Christopher Columbus may have had reactive arthritis, this is speculative. It was first noted associated with venereal disease at the end of the eighteenth century. These disorders were often "rediscovered". There are several good examples from the 1914–1918 European war. In 1916, two French physicians, Fiessinger and Leroy described four cases of conjunctivitis and arthritis after diarrhoeal illness. The same year Reiter reported a young officer in the Balkan front who after acute diarrhoea developed arthritis, urethritis and conjunctivitis.

Diagnosis

The Concept of Classification Criteria

There are no diagnostic criteria for any of the inflammatory arthropathies. This is because there is no single test by which any of the diseases can be definitively diagnosed. Classification criteria however exist, which provide a standardised approach for identifying individuals with a high probability of having a disease for enrolment into research studies. They are often used in clinical practice to aid diagnosis although the gold standard remains the opinion of an experienced rheumatologist.

Rheumatoid Arthritis

It is usually straightforward to diagnose RA. Sometimes it can be problematic, particularly when there are non-specific presenting features. One difficulty is the absence of definitive laboratory tests and confirmatory physical findings in early disease. For the last few decades the internationally accepted classification criteria was the 1987 American College of Rheumatology (ACR) criteria [1]. According to these RA is considered to be present when 4 of 7 qualifying criteria are met (Table 1.1).

Although these criteria have high overall sensitivity and specificity, because they were developed from patients with established RA they lack accuracy in diagnosing RA in its early stages. They therefore have limited value in distinguishing new-onset RA from a self-limiting arthritis. The last few years have seen a major change in the paradigm of RA treatment towards early diagnosis and prompt intensive treatment. The RA classification criteria were therefore recently updated in 2010 by a joint working group of the ACR and European League Against Rheumatism (EULAR) to facilitate the early identification of RA [2]. These new criteria classify the presence of RA based on synovitis in at least 1 joint, the absence of an alternative diagnosis and the achievement of a total score of at least 6 (from a possible score of 10) from marks across four domains (Table 1.1).

Ankylosing Spondylitis

AS is often considered to be the main spondyloarthritis. Its predominant features are in the spine, with evidence of spinal inflammation that focuses on the sacroiliac joints, termed sacroiliitis. Other features include evidence of inflammation at the insertion of tendons into bone – termed enthesitis. Finally a minority of patients have a large joint peripheral arthritis. Conventional classification criteria focus on spinal symptoms and x-ray features of sacroiliitis, the most

TABLE 1.1 Comparison of 1987 and 2010 criteria for classifying rheumatoid arthritis

1987 American College of Rheumatology Criteria for classifying RA	2010 American College of Rheumatology/European League Against Rheumatism Classification Criteria for RA
1. Morning stiffness lasting longer than 1 h before improvement	Definite clinical synovitis (swelling) of at least 1 joint *and* Synovitis not better explained by another pathology *and* Score of ≥6/10 from the following four domains:
2. Arthritis involving three or more joint areas	1. Joint involvement
	1 large joint = 0 points
	2–10 large joints = 1 point
	1–3 small joints = 2 points
	4–10 small joints = 3 points
	>10 joints (at least 1 small joint) = 5 points
3. Arthritis of the hand joints	2. Serology
	Negative RF and negative ACPA = 0 points
	Low-positive RF or low-positive ACPA = 2 points
	High-positive RF or high-positive ACPA = 3 points

3. Acute-phase response

Normal CRP and ESR = 0 points

Abnormal CRP or ESR = 1 point

4. Duration of symptoms

<6 weeks = 0 points

≥6 weeks = 1 point

4. Symmetrical arthritis

5. Rheumatoid nodules

6. Positive serum RF

7. Radiographic evidence of RA

To diagnose RA criteria 1–4 must have been present for at least 6 weeks; 4 or more criteria must be present. The diagnosis of RA should not be made by criteria alone if another systemic disease associated with arthritis is definitely present

To diagnose RA patients must satisfy all three criteria. Low positive serological tests refer to values ≤3 times the upper limit of normal; high positive refers to values >3 times the upper limit of normal. RF = Rheumatoid Factor; ACPA = Antibodies to Citrullinated Protein Antigens

Table adapted from 1987 ACR and 2010 ACR/EULAR RA classification criteria [1, 2]

TABLE 1.2 Modified New York criteria for classifying ankylosing spondylitis

Clinical features	Radiological changes
Limited movement of lumbar spine in three planes	Severe (grade 3–4) unilateral sacroiliitis *or* moderate (grade 2) bilateral sacroiliitis
Inflammatory lower back pain	
Reduced chest expansion	

Table based on Modified New York classification criteria reported by van der Linden et al. [3]
Inflammatory back pain is defined as lower back pain for ≥3 months, improved by exercise and not relieved by rest. To be classified with definite AS at least one clinical and radiological criterion must be fulfilled

established of which is the 1984 modified New York criteria (Table 1.2) [3]. This requires the patient to have sacroillitis on plain X-rays alongside clinical features of inflammatory spinal pain and/or restricted spinal or thoracic cage movement.

The predominant problem with the modified New York classification criteria is that it can take several years for sacroiliitis to develop on plain X-ray. The criteria therefore lack sensitivity in early disease with some patients taking up to 8 years from disease onset to fulfil the criteria by which point they may have significant spinal fusion. This has led to the development of updated criteria, which have been validated in the Assessment of Spondyloarthritis International Society (ASAS) study [4]. These criteria include patients with and without radiographic changes and focus on sacroiliitis seen on magnetic resonance imaging (MRI), which can be seen early on in the disease process (Table 1.3). MRI sacroiliitis has a close correlation with the later appearance of sacroiliitis on plain radiographs and has an estimated sensitivity and specificity of 90 %.

TABLE 1.3 Assessment of Spondyloarthritis International Society (ASAS) classification criteria for axial spondyloarthritis [4]

Radiological criteria	Genetic criteria
Radiographic or MRI evidence of sacroiliitis AND ≥1 spondyloarthritis feature	Presence of HLA-B27 AND ≥2 spondyloarthritis features

Patients are classified as having an axial spondyloarthritis if they have back pain of ≥3 months duration and age of symptom onset <45 years and meet the radiological or genetic criteria

Spondyloarthritis features comprise inflammatory back pain, arthritis, enthesitis (heel), uveitis, dactylitis, psoriasis, inflammatory bowel disease, good NSAID response, familial history of spondyloarthritis, HLA-B27 positive, raised CRP

Psoriatic Arthritis

There has been less agreement on the criteria for classifying PsA compared with other common forms of inflammatory arthritis. The Moll and Wright classification criteria have often been applied, which require patients to have an inflammatory arthritis, psoriasis and to usually be seronegative for RF [5]. They divide patients into five subgroups based on their pattern of joint involvement, which comprise distal interphalangeal (DIP) joint arthritis, asymmetrical oligoarthritis, polyarthritis, spondylitis and arthritis mutilans. These criteria lack specificity with a proportion of patients that fulfil the criteria for psoriatic polyarthritis probably having RA with coincidental psoriasis.

More recently the classification criteria for PsA (CASPAR) criteria have been introduced (Fig. 1.1) [6]. These are gaining acceptance as a useful diagnostic tool in clinical practice. To fulfil these criteria patients must have inflammatory articular disease (either of the joint, spine or entheseal) and score ≥3 points from five separate categories comprising past medical or familial evidence of psoriasis, characteristic nail changes, a

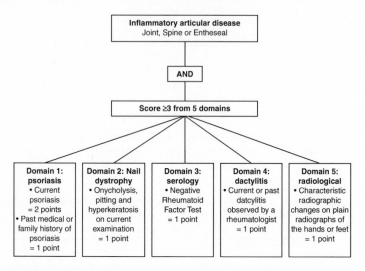

FIGURE 1.1 The Classification Criteria for PsA (CASPAR) criteria (Taylor et al. [6]

negative RF, dactylitis or characteristic radiological changes. These criteria have a sensitivity of 91 % and specificity of 99 %. They recognise the fact that in a proportion of cases PsA can precede the onset of skin disease and therefore do not require psoriasis to be present in order to be classified as having PsA.

Other Spondyloarthropathies

There is less agreement on the criteria for diagnosing reactive arthritis, enteropathic arthritis and undifferentiated seronegative arthropathies. Reactive arthritis is usually considered present in patients with an inflammatory peripheral joint oligoarthritis or axial arthritis and a recent episode of gastroenteritis caused by *Shigella, Salmonella, Campylobacter,* or *Yersinia*, or genitourinary tract infection with *Chlamydia trachomatis*. Enteropathic arthritis is considered present in patients with features of a spondyloarthritis in the context of diagnosed IBD.

References

1. Arnett FC, Edworthy SM, Bloch DA, McShane DJ, Fries JF, Cooper NS, et al. The American Rheumatism Association 1987 revised criteria for the classification of rheumatoid arthritis. Arthritis Rheum. 1988;31:315–24.
2. Aletaha D, Neogi T, Silman AJ, Funovits J, Felson DT, Bingham 3rd CO, et al. 2010 rheumatoid arthritis classification criteria: an American College of Rheumatology/European League Against Rheumatism collaborative initiative. Arthritis Rheum. 2010;62:2569–81.
3. van der Linden S, Valkenburg HA, Cats A. Evaluation of diagnostic criteria for ankylosing spondylitis. A proposal for modification of the New York criteria. Arthritis Rheum. 1984;27:361–8.
4. Rudwaleit M, van der Heijde D, Landewe R, Listing J, Akkoc N, Brandt J, et al. The development of Assessment of SpondyloArthritis international Society classification criteria for axial spondyloarthritis (part II): validation and final selection. Ann Rheum Dis. 2009;68:777–83.
5. Moll JM, Wright V. Psoriatic arthritis. Semin Arthritis Rheum. 1973;3:55–78.
6. Taylor W, Gladman D, Helliwell P, Marchesoni A, Mease P, Mielants H, et al. Classification criteria for psoriatic arthritis: development of new criteria from a large international study. Arthritis Rheum. 2006;54:2665–73.

Chapter 2
Epidemiology and Pathology

Abstract RA and the seronegative spondyloarthropathies are relatively common disorders with a prevalence of approximately 1 % in European and North American populations. They are complex diseases that are considered to result from environmental exposures in genetically predisposed individuals. The main genetic risk factors are in the HLA region, with *HLA-DRB1* and *HLA-B27* alleles being the dominant risk factors for RA and AS, respectively. Environmental factors play an important role in RA development, particularly exposure to cigarette smoke. A broad range of immune system components are involved in the precipitation and perpetuation of the inflammatory arthropathies, particularly cytokines such as tumour necrosis factor-α. This chapter will provide an overview of the epidemiology of the inflammatory arthropathies, their underlying genetic and environmental risk factors, alongside the immunopathological changes that characterise them.

Keywords Prevalence • Complex Disease • HLA Risk • Cigarette Smoking • Cytokines

I.C. Scott et al., *Inflammatory Arthritis in Clinical Practice*,
DOI 10.1007/978-1-4471-6648-1_2,
© Springer-Verlag London 2015

Epidemiology of Rheumatoid Arthritis

Although RA is an international problem, there is a wide geographical variation in its prevalence. It is relatively common in European and North American populations, with a widely quoted prevalence (the proportion of individuals with the disease at any given time) of 1 % in the UK. By contrast the disease is much rarer in developing countries such as Nigeria and Pakistan where its prevalence is estimated at less than 0.5 % [1]. These variations probably reflect differences in genetic risks and environmental exposures. There is some evidence that the prevalence of RA is changing. A seminal study by Lawrence in 1961 found a prevalence of RA in two Northern UK areas of 1 % [2]. A more recent study in 2002 of the Norfolk population estimated the adult prevalence of RA to be 0.81 % [3]. Comparing the prevalence of RA in the Lawrence and Norfolk studies stratified by age group and gender suggests the fall in prevalence is confined to women (Fig. 2.1).

The age distribution of RA is unimodal with a peak incidence between the fourth and sixth decade. Compared to men, women are two to three times more likely to develop RA. As RA is a chronic disease the incidence of new cases is relatively rare.

Epidemiology of Seronegative Arthritis

There is a strong association between seronegative arthritis and *HLA-B27*. The presence of this genotype and male sex are dominant factors in the epidemiology of seronegative arthritis. The prevalence of spondyloarthropathies in European and North American white populations may be as high as 1.5 %, though most experts consider it is below 1 %. There is an excess of males in almost all subsets of spondyloarthropathy. Geographical variation in the prevalence of spondyloarthropathies reflects variations in the number of people who are *HLA-B27* positive. AS and undifferentiated

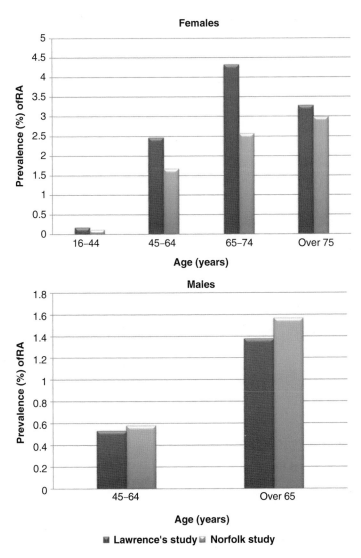

FIGURE 2.1 Comparing the prevalence of rheumatoid arthritis from two studies Undertaken in 1961 (Lawrence Study) and 2002 (Norfolk Study) (Figure adapted using data reported by Lawrence [2] and Symmons et al. [3])

spondyloarthropathy are the most frequent spondyloarthropathy subtypes. Individuals with inflammatory back pain who are *HLA-B27* positive have a 50 % likelihood of having sacroiliitis.

Aetiology of Inflammatory Arthritis

The inflammatory arthropathies are considered to be complex disorders that occur when genetically predisposed individuals are exposed to environmental factors. These gene-environment risk factors interact causing changes in the immune system and a subsequent inflammatory arthritis.

Rheumatoid Arthritis

Genetic and environmental risk factors are best defined for RA, particularly the subtype in which autoantibodies – RF or antibodies to citrullinated protein antigens (ACPA) – are present, termed seropositive RA. Most genetic risk for seropositive RA is derived from the HLA region, specifically a group of alleles called *HLA-DRB1*. These encode the HLA class II DRβ-chain, which plays a vital role in the presentation of antigens to T cells. *HLA-DRB1* alleles encoding a group of amino acid sequences (QRRAA, RRRAA and QKRAA) spanning positions 70–74 of the HLA-DRβ1 molecule particularly increase the risk of seropositive RA [4]. These alleles are known as the shared epitope (SE) alleles. A recent large analysis combining genetic studies of patients with and without RA has identified 100 genetic markers that predispose to RA development that are external to the HLA region [5].

The main environmental risk factor for seropositive RA is smoking. A dose-response relationship is seen, whereby the risk of RA increases as more cigarettes are smoked over time. This risk is especially increased in individuals carrying SE alleles. Other environmental risk factors include alcohol abstinence, nulliparity and a history of never breast-feeding.

Seronegative Spondyloarthropathies

The dominant genetic risk factor for the seronegative spondyloarthropathies is *HLA-B27*. This is particularly true in AS, with most AS populations studied having *HLA-B27* present in over 80 % of individuals [6]. However, carrying this allele does not mean that AS will develop, with less than 5 % of *HLA-B27* carriers developing AS [6].

With the exception of the role that genitourinary or gastrointestinal infections play in triggering a reactive arthritis, environmental risk factors for the seronegative spondyloarthropathies are less well defined when compared with RA. Whilst it has long been postulated that an infectious agent may trigger these conditions through interactions with *HLA-B27* no single microbe has been identified consistently across patient populations. A recent population-based study suggests that obesity is associated with an increased risk of PsA [7].

Pathology of Inflammatory Arthritis

Histology

Inflammatory synovitis is the key pathological feature in RA. Its characteristics are synovial hyperplasia, inflammatory cell infiltration and vascularity. Initially oedema and fibrin deposition predominate. Subsequently there is synovial lining layer hyperplasia involving macrophage-like and fibroblast-like synoviocytes. This hyperplasia is accompanied by infiltration of T cells, B cells, macrophages and plasma cells in the sublining layer. Endothelial cells in the blood vessels transform to form high endothelial venules.

Pannus formation, with the formation of locally invasive synovial tissue, is the other characteristic feature of RA. It underlies cartilage damage and joint erosions. The RA pannus is composed of mononuclear cells and fibroblasts. It has high levels of proteolytic enzyme expression, which allows

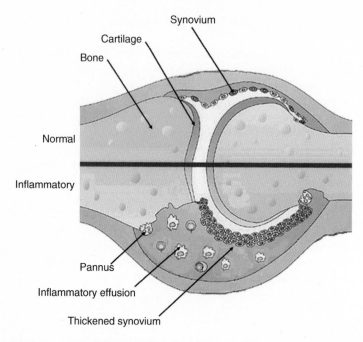

FIGURE 2.2 Normal and inflamed synovium in inflammatory arthritis

the pannus to penetrate cartilage. In late RA the pannus becomes fibrotic, with minimally vascularised pannus and collagen fibres overlying articular cartilage. These changes are shown in Fig. 2.2.

Lymphocytes

Many inflammatory cells in the synovial sublining layer are lymphocytes, especially T cells. They sometimes form aggregates like those of lymph nodes. Despite the presence of many T cells in the RA synovium, these T cells probably do not directly cause synovitis in the microenvironment of the joint. Instead there appears to be recruitment of previously stimulated, mature T cells into the joint.

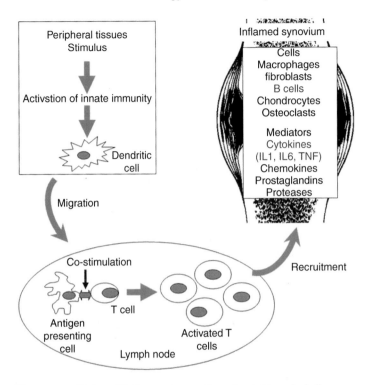

FIGURE 2.3 Roles of inflammatory cells and cytokines in inflammatory arthritis

Cytokines

Cytokines are small soluble proteins involved in communication between cells participating in immune responses. They mediate cell division, differentiation and chemotaxis. Some cytokines are pro-inflammatory and others are anti-inflammatory. Two cytokines – tumour necrosis factor-alpha (TNF-α) and interleukin-1 – are present in large quantities in RA synovial fluid and tissue. These cytokines have become therapeutic targets. The roles of cytokines and inflammatory cells are shown in Fig. 2.3.

Chemokines

These small chemoattractant proteins have prominent roles in leukocyte recruitment and activation at inflammatory sites. Numerous chemokines are active in RA synovium, though their functions are not fully elucidated.

Metalloproteinases

High levels of these destructive enzymes are produced by RA synovial lining cells. There is a large family of matrix metalloproteinase enzymes. They are involved in remodelling and destruction of the extracellular matrix and articular cartilage. Their activities are modulated by tissue inhibitors of metalloproteinases, serine proteinase inhibitors and α2-macroglobulin.

Adhesion Molecules, Angiogenesis and Other Mediators

Adhesion molecules are involved in recruitment of inflammatory cells in RA. They enable cells to adhere both to each other and to the extracellular matrix. Expression of adhesion molecules in synovial tissue contributes to the recruitment and retention of inflammatory cells. Angiogenesis, the formation of new blood vessels, is active in RA, particularly the early stages. Newly formed vessels are needed to sustain the hypertrophied synovium. It is regulated by many inducers and inhibitors. These include cytokines, growth factors and soluble adhesion molecules. RA synovitis is mediated by many other enzymes including cyclo-oxygenases, nitric oxide synthase and neutral proteases. Their precise roles are uncertain.

References

1. Kalla AA, Tikly M. Rheumatoid arthritis in the developing world. Best Pract Res Clin Rheumatol. 2003;17:863–75.

2. Lawrence JS. Prevalence of rheumatoid arthritis. Ann Rheum Dis. 1961;20:11–7.
3. Symmons D, Turner G, Webb R, Asten P, Barrett E, Lunt M, et al. The prevalence of rheumatoid arthritis in the United Kingdom: new estimates for a new century. Rheumatology (Oxford). 2002; 41:793–800.
4. Gregersen PK, Silver J, Winchester RJ. The shared epitope hypothesis. An approach to understanding the molecular genetics of susceptibility to rheumatoid arthritis. Arthritis Rheum. 1987;30:1205–13.
5. Okada Y, Wu D, Trynka G, Towfique R, Chikashi T, Katsunori I, et al. Genetics of rheumatoid arthritis contributes to biology and drug discovery. Nat Genet. 2013;506:376–81.
6. Brown MA. Genetics of ankylosing spondylitis. Curr Opin Rheumatol. 2010;22:126–32.
7. Love TJ, Zhu Y, Zhang Y, Wall-Burns L, Ogdie A, Gelfand JM, et al. Obesity and the risk of psoriatic arthritis: a population-based study. Ann Rheum Dis. 2012;71:1273–7.

Chapter 3
Clinical Features

Abstract   The hallmark of the inflammatory arthropathies is joint inflammation, characterised by joint pain and swelling. Different disease types affect different joints. RA classically affects the peripheral small joints in a symmetrical fashion. By contrast the seronegative spondyloarthropathies tend to affect the spine and peripheral large joints in an asymmetrical fashion. Extra-articular features are common in all forms of inflammatory arthritis. In RA almost any body system can be affected, with manifestations ranging from rheumatoid nodules to mononeuritis multiplex. The classical extra-articular manifestation of the seronegative spondyloarthropathies is anterior uveitis. This chapter will discuss the clinical manifestations of the inflammatory arthropathies, spanning their articular and extra-articular features.

Keywords   Synovitis • Tenosynovitis • Tender Joints • Enthesitis • Extra-Articular Involvement

I.C. Scott et al., *Inflammatory Arthritis in Clinical Practice*,
DOI 10.1007/978-1-4471-6648-1_3,
© Springer-Verlag London 2015

Synovitis of Peripheral Joints

Symptoms

The main symptoms of inflammatory arthritis result from inflammation of the joints. Pain is a dominant symptom both within the joints and more diffusely around the joints. The joints are also swollen and tender and they are difficult to move.

The symptoms often show diurnal variation. Patients have most problems early in the morning. As a result they usually have prolonged morning stiffness. This can last up to several hours. It usually lasts over 30 minutes. The exact nature of the stiffness can be difficult to define and not all patients describe it in the same manner.

Joint Swelling and Tenderness

The characteristic features of inflamed joints are swelling and tenderness [1]. Joint swelling is soft tissue swelling detected along joint margins. When there is a synovial effusion, a joint is inevitably swollen. However, effusions are not mandatory features of a swollen joint. The characteristic feature of a swollen joint is fluctuation, when fluid is displaced by pressure in two planes.

Bony swelling and joint deformities often complicate the counting of swollen joints. Neither of these indicates the presence of joint swelling, although they can be present if joints are swollen. In late disease it is often difficult to differentiate swollen from deformed inactive joints.

An associated clinical feature that accompanies joint swelling is swelling of tendon sheaths – termed tenosynovitis. It involves an identical pathological process.

Joint tenderness is indicated by inducing pain in a joint at rest with pressure. Judging the correct amount of pressure to elicit tenderness depends on both the examiner and the patient. Generally sufficient pressure should be exerted by the examiner's thumb and index finger to cause 'whitening' of the examiner's nail bed. Too little pressure may fail to elicit joint tenderness even though it is present. Too much pressure will result in pain in everyone. The level of pressure required to elicit joint tenderness varies from one patient to another. In some joints, like the hip, tenderness is best identified through movement.

Peripheral Joints Involved

RA is usually a symmetrical polyarthritis. It mainly involves the hand, wrists, feet, and some large joints, particularly the knees. In some patients it only involves a few joints at the outset, though more become involved over time [2, 3].

Other forms of inflammatory arthritis usually involve fewer joints. The distribution of joint involvement is also less obviously symmetrical [4]. Each form of inflammatory arthritis has its own relatively characteristic distribution of joint involvement.

Rheumatoid Arthritis

Hand involvement is particularly characteristic of RA (Fig. 3.1). It usually involves the metacarpophalangeal, proximal interphalangeal, thumb interphalangeal and wrist joints. The distal interphalangeal joints can be affected when there is coexisting disease in other hand joints.

Involvement of the tendons is also characteristic. Tenosynovitis of flexor tendons reduces finger flexion and strength. Nodular thickenings in tendon sheaths may result in a trigger finger.

Damage to the wrists causes compaction of bone at the small wrist joints. In late disease this damage may progress to bony ankylosis. Historically in late RA characteristic deformities developed in the hands. There was ulnar deviation of the fingers, subluxation of the metacarpophalangeal joints, hyperextension of the proximal interphalangeal with flexion of the distal joints (swan-neck deformity), flexion of the

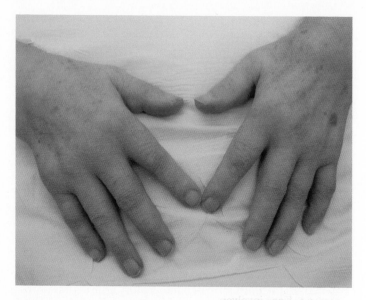

FIGURE 3.1 An inflamed hand in early rheumatoid arthritis

proximal interphalangeal with hyperextension of the distal joints (boutonnière deformity), and a Z-shaped deformity of the thumb. These changes are seen less often in the modern era.

The small joints of the feet are involved at an early stage, causing considerable difficulty walking. As the disease progresses a complex series of changes occurs in the feet including spreading of the forefoot, dorsal subluxation of toes and subluxation of metatarsal heads to a subcutaneous site on the plantar surface. In some cases additional hallux valgus leads to "stacking" of the second and third toes on top of the great toe.

The ankle joint itself is rarely involved in RA, although it is sometimes damaged in late disease. By contrast the subtalar joint is often involved. Its involvement results in pronation deformities and eversion of the foot. The reason for such a different level of involvement in adjacent joint is most likely the effects of microtrauma on the severity of synovitis. The ankle is in a relatively atraumatic environment compared to the subtalar joint.

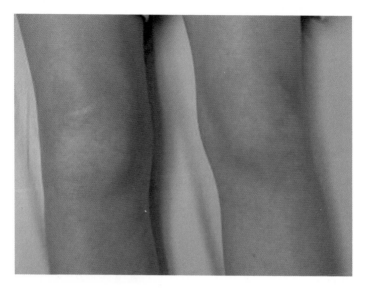

FIGURE 3.2 Knee involvement in rheumatoid arthritis

Knee involvement is common in RA including both early and late disease. Quadriceps wasting and loss of full extension both occur in the first stages of the disease.

In some patients there may be large effusions (Fig. 3.2), and these can result in a popliteal or Baker's cyst. Synovial fluid entering these popliteal cysts does not readily return into the knee. One consequence is that high pressures may be generated and the cyst can rupture into the calf, resulting in considerable pain and discomfort.

RA often affects the synovium of the glenohumeral joint in the shoulder and its associated bursae. In addition it involves the rotator cuff together with its associated muscles on the chest wall. Weakness of the rotator cuff apparatus may result in shoulder subluxation.

The hips are rarely involved in the early stages of RA. However, their involvement is more frequent in late disease. Eventually about half of rheumatoid patients develop some evidence of hip disease. About 20 % of patients develop significant levels of hip pain with resulting joint failure.

In a small number of patients the femoral head collapses. The acetabulum is remodelled and pushed medially. This results in protrusio acetabuli. The deformity usually progresses until the femoral neck impinges on side of pelvis.

Cervical pain is common in the early phases of RA. This pain is mainly due to muscle spasm. However, over the subsequent course of their disease up to 90 % of patients develop some cervical spine involvement. The likelihood of severe cervical spine involvement is increased in long standing disease and when many joints are involved. Significant subluxations occur in about one third of cases. Neurological deterioration can be irreversible in such cases, and it is therefore important to look for subtle signs of early neurological involvement. In addition to painful limitation of neck motion, warning signs of significant cervical involvement include sub-occipital pain, paraesthesia in hands and feet, urinary retention and incontinence and involuntary leg spasms.

Psoriatic Arthritis

PsA has highly variable clinical features and there are several different patterns of joint involvement [5]. These tend to change over time.

Conventionally PsA is divided into five different clinical subtypes. These clinical subtypes comprise:

1. Polyarthritis: many joints are involved and the clinical pattern is very similar to RA
2. Oligoarthritis: in most patients with PsA only two or three joints are involved. As a consequence the arthritis seems very asymmetric.
3. Monoarthritis: as the classification indicates only one joint is involved. Over time the pattern may change with the involvement of more joints.
4. Distal interphalangeal joint arthritis: this is a highly characteristic arthritis of the distal interphalangeal joints of the hands. It can be very destructive.

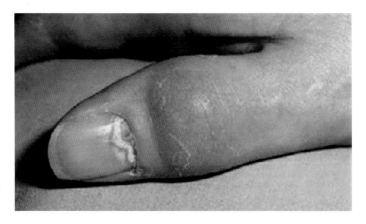

FIGURE 3.3 Psoriatic arthritis involving the thumb joint

5. Arthritis mutilans: this is the rare but highly progressive and destructive form of arthritis which is seen in occasional patients (Fig. 3.3).

Other Forms of Spondyloarthropathies

Peripheral joint inflammation can be the presenting feature in many patients with a spondyloarthritis. It can also occur against the background of established inflammatory back disease in AS.

In these seronegative types of arthritis usually only one or two joints are involved. Patients have an oligoarthritis, which is mainly seen in lower limbs. It is usually asymmetric in distribution. The most commonly involved joints are the knees. In some patients the elbows can also be involved.

Enthesitis

The entheses are the insertion of tendons into bone [6]. These are frequently inflamed in spondyloarthritis. Such inflammation is known as an enthesitis. It involves sites such as the insertion of the Achilles tendon – Achilles tendonitis – and insertion of the plantar fascia – plantar fasciitis. Other sites involved include the greater trochanters, the pelvic brim, and the epicondyles.

In addition some patients with PsA have a dactylitis, which is colloquially termed "sausage" fingers. This is a more diffuse inflammatory change than either arthritis or enthesitis and is typical of PsA.

Spinal Disease

Involvement of the sacroiliac joints, other cartilaginous joints like the pubic symphysis, and the spine is the central feature of AS and other seronegative spondyloarthropathies [7]. It is less common, and very different, in RA.

Ankylosing Spondylitis

AS usually starts with back pain and stiffness of insidious onset. It mainly affects males and begins in late adolescence and early adult life. These symptoms reflect the combination of sacroiliac joint and spinal disease. There is spinal pain and stiffness and loss of mobility. These symptoms are usually intermittent in the early stages of the disease. They reflect both spinal inflammation and structural damage. Inflammation includes spondylitis, spondylodiscitis and spondyloarthritis. The structural changes are usually due to oestoproliferation rather than destruction. Ankylosis and syndesmophytes are characteristic findings.

In the early stages of AS the pain may be a dull ache in the buttock region, which reflects involvement of the sacroiliac joints. Initially it may be unilateral or intermittent. However, over time it becomes persistent and bilateral. There may be accompanying sacroiliac and spinal tenderness. In some patients low back pain can be minimal. Occasionally pain is more marked in the thoracic or cervical spine.

In late disease the whole spine may be involved with pain and reduced movement. Spinal fusion is a serious, though relatively uncommon, consequence of persisting spinal inflammation in AS.

Anterior chest wall pain, reflecting involvement of the manubriosternal joints and other joints, is relatively common in AS but is often overlooked as a clinical problem. It affects about one third of patients to a greater or lesser extent.

Other Types of Spondyloarthritis

PsA, reactive arthritis, IBD-related or enteropathic arthritis and undifferentiated spondyloarthritis can all have an element of inflammatory back changes as part of their clinical spectrum. This is broadly similar to the findings in AS, though less severe.

Rheumatoid Arthritis

The cervical spine is often involved in RA [8], as there are a number of important synovial joints at this site. As a result cervical instability is an important clinical problem, though it only affects a minority of patients to any great extent. The rest of the spine is not specifically affected by RA, though occasional patients may have facet joint disease. Patients with RA may have back pain in the same way as the general population.

Systemic Features

Arthritis causes general ill health in addition to the synovitis. Patients feel tired and lack energy. They also often have systemic features of a "flu-like" illness. These include loss of appetite, inability to sleep, some weight loss and, in some cases a low-grade fever. These systemic features are most noticeable at the onset of arthritis, especially in cases with an explosive onset. It is likely they represent the non-specific inflammatory response of immunity.

Fatigue is closely associated with pain and systemic involvement in arthritis. It is not directly related to the arthritis, but is has a major impact on patient well-being and health status.

Clinical Course

Onset of Rheumatoid Arthritis

Most patients have an insidious onset [9]. They develop features of arthritis over weeks or months. Their initial symptoms may be systemic, articular or both. Some cases initially describe fatigue, malaise, puffy hands and diffuse joint pain, with joints becoming involved later. In 5–10 % there is an acute onset with the "explosive" beginning of symptoms over a few days. Some patients pinpoint the onset of symptoms to a specific time or activity. Symptoms rapidly progress over several days or weeks and there may be marked systemic symptoms. Between these extremes about 20 % have an intermediate onset over days and weeks.

Occasional patients have atypical onsets. Examples include palindromic, polymyalgic and monoarticular onsets. Cases with polymyalgic onsets present with shoulder girdle pain and prolonged morning stiffness.

By contrast palindromic rheumatism can be the initial manifestation of many different rheumatic disorders organic processes, and may never evolve into significant disease. It is characterised by pain, which usually begins in one joint or in periarticular tissues. Symptoms worsen for several hours or days and are associated with swelling. Then symptoms resolve without any residual. In some cases this pattern gradually transforms into typical RA [10].

Finally a few cases present with either a monoarticular onset or an asymmetric pattern of disease, usually involving the knee joints. This is seen in about 10–20 % of cases, but usually progresses into the more typical polyarticular pattern of RA.

Established Rheumatoid Arthritis

RA is usually considered to have three different courses [11]. Most patients have a progressive course. These patients have persistent joint inflammation, progressive joint damage and gradual increases in disability. However there can be major fluctuations in disease severity over time and not all patients show inexorable progression.

A minority of patients have intermittent disease courses. These patients have intermittent episodes of arthritis, which may last less than 1 year, followed by variable remissions. These remissions can be brief or they may be long-lasting. With modern intensive treatment more patients are achieving remission and having more intermittent disease courses.

Occasional patients have what has been termed "malignant disease". They have severe progressive arthritis which is often accompanied by major extra-articular problems. It has a potentially serious outcome, though modern intensive treatment is usually able to control it.

Other Inflammatory Arthropathies

The other forms of inflammatory arthritis have similar onsets to RA. They can develop suddenly or insidiously. However, there are some important differences. Unlike RA they are usually less severe and often enter remission.

Undifferentiated Early Arthritis

In the first few months or longer after the development of an inflammatory arthritis it can be difficult to tell whether a patient has early RA or another, potentially less severe form of inflammatory arthritis. These patients are considered to have an "undifferentiated" arthritis. It is usually best to consider they are likely to develop into RA as watchful waiting may be unhelpful in that it will result in the risk of under-treatment.

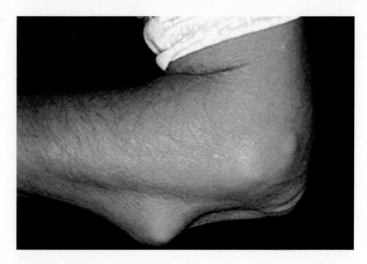

Figure 3.4 Rheumatoid nodules

Extra-articular Disease

Rheumatoid Arthritis

Between 20 and 40 % of cases have extra-articular features of
RA [12]. These are most prominent in seropositive patients
with high RF titres. The extra-articular features vary in severity and duration, and only cause major problems in a few
cases. However, much of the morbidity and excess mortality
of RA is concentrated in patients with extra-articular disease.

Rheumatoid nodules are the most characteristic extra-
articular feature of RA (Fig. 3.4). They are subcutaneous nodules of varying size from 5 mm to several centimetres. Nodules
effect about one quarter of cases. They are mainly seen in seropositive disease. Most are subcutaneous on extensor surfaces
like the olecranon process. They vary in consistency from soft
mobile masses to hard, rubbery masses attached to underlying
periosteum. Atypical nodules can be confusing; for example
sacral nodules may be confused with bedsores if the overlying

skin breaks down. Sometimes nodules cause local problems, for example nodules in heart valves can precipitate heart failure. They do not usually require treatment, unless they ulcerate or compress nerves. They may regress with standard therapy though sometimes they persist or worsen during treatment. Occasional patients treated with methotrexate develop accelerated rheumatoid nodulosis. In these patients multiple small nodules develop in the fingers and hands.

Rheumatoid vasculitis is the other most characteristic extra-articular feature of RA. Many of the other extra-articular features of the disease can be viewed as being an expression of rheumatoid vasculitis. About 1–5 % of patients develop rheumatoid vasculitis. Its frequency is declining over time. It mainly affects seropositive patients. Rheumatoid vasculitis can affect any organ. However, most cases have cutaneous features. These include focal digital ischemia, deep cutaneous ulcers, petecchiae, purpura and peripheral gangrene. Isolated digital vasculitis, with characteristic splinter-lesions around nails, is a marker of severe disease that rarely causes problems itself. By contrast systemic vasculitis can be a devastating complication involving internal organs such as the bowel. Vasculitis classically occurs in "burned-out" RA patients with nodular and RF-positive destructive disease that is no longer active. Occasionally vasculitis complicates early disease.

Neurological problems can involve both peripheral and central nervous systems. They are often attributed to vasculitis affecting the vasa vasorum of nerves leading to ischemic damage. This vasculitis of the blood vessels of nerves results in neurovascular disease, which ranges from a mild sensory neuropathy to a severe sensorimotor neuropathy. In some patients there is a mononeuritis multiplex, in which a number of different peripheral nerves become damaged. Central nervous system vasculitis has been described but is extremely rare. Local compression of peripheral nerves, particularly as part of carpal tunnel syndrome is, by comparison, very common. Finally cervical myelopathy due to atlanto-axial subluxation occurs in occasional patients with long-standing disease. It is due to a combination of local synovitis and bone deformity.

A range of eye problems can occur. These include secondary Sjögren's syndrome, episcleritis, scleritis, keratitis and retinopathy. Anterior scleritis can be diffuse, nodular or necrotizing; this latter condition is also known as scleromalacia perforans. It involves degenerative thinning of the sclera and if not treated can lead to scleral perforation.

Lung problems are common in RA [13]. Depending on how they are classified they can affect 10–25 % of patients. They result in considerable morbidity. They are highly variable problems. They include interstitial lung disease, small airway disease, rheumatoid nodules, pleural effusion and pulmonary vasculitis. Some patients with RA have coexisting bronchiectasis. Patients with RA who smoke cigarettes are more likely to have lung problems and their severity is likely to be greater.

Cardiac disorders are also relatively common in RA [14]. All parts of the heart can be involved. Patients can have pericarditis, myocarditis, valvular disease and conduction defects and arrhythmias. There is also an increased risk of ischemic heart disease. In addition hypertension is relatively common in RA, though how much this reflects the disease and how much is due to its treatment is uncertain. Symptomatic pericarditis affects about 1–5 % of patients, and is particularly common in seropositive men with RA.

Skin involvement includes palmar erythema, pyoderma gangrenosum, vasculitic rashes and leg ulceration. Occasional patients have Felty's syndrome (low white cell counts with splenomegaly) or amyloid deposits.

Other Inflammatory Arthropathies

The spectrum of extra-articular disease is strikingly different in the seronegative spondyloarthropathies compared to RA [15]. Some of the extra-articular features in the spondyloarthropathies are part of the main diagnostic categorisation. Patients with PsA have psoriasis. Patients with enteropathic arthritis have IBD. Patients with reactive arthritis have urethritis or diarrhoea.

Some of these condition-specific problems are seen in other disorders of this group. For example, psoriasis may be seen in reactive arthritis, when patients develop psoriatic changes in the skin of their hands and feet. These changes are termed keratoderma blenhoragicum. Another example is the development of balanitis. The reaction overlaps with psoriatic changes involving the glans penis. It is termed circinate balanitis. It can occur together with urethritis, though this latter problem has a different clinical course.

Inflammatory eye involvement is a relatively common and potentially serious problem. Acute anterior uveitis occurs in about 30 % of patients with spondyloarthritis. Its clinical course is not directly related to the rheumatic condition. In some patients eye inflammation precedes the spondylitis. Anterior uveitis causes pain, redness of the eye and photophobia. Its onset is usually acute. Conjunctivitis, episcleritis and scleritis can all also occur in spondyloarthropathies. As eye inflammation, particularly if it is recurrent, can lead to visual loss, patients with this complication need prompt specialist ophthalmic management.

Cardiac disease is seen in many patients with seronegative spondyloarthritis. It is usually ischaemic heart disease and hypertension, related to active inflammation, treatment and smoking. A minority of patient have cardiac conduction defects. An unusual but rare feature is aortic valve disease in AS, which may result in aortic valve incompetence.

In longstanding spinal disease there may be chest wall rigidity. This may impair lung function. Occasionally patients with AS can present with upper zone pulmonary fibrosis. Other chest problems include sleep apnoea and the development of a spontaneous pneumothorax.

References

1. van der Heijde DM, van 't Hof MA, van Riel PL, Theunisse LA, Lubberts EW, van Leeuwen MA, et al. Judging disease activity in clinical practice in rheumatoid arthritis: first step in the development of a disease activity score. Ann Rheum Dis. 1990;49:916–20.

2. Scott DL, Wolfe F, Huizinga TW. Rheumatoid arthritis. Lancet. 2010;376:1094–108.
3. Klarenbeek NB, Kerstens PJ, Huizinga TW, Dijkmans BA, Allaart CF. Recent advances in the management of rheumatoid arthritis. BMJ. 2010;341:c6942.
4. Helliwell PS, Hetthen J, Sokoll K, Green M, Marchesoni A, Lubrano E, et al. Joint symmetry in early and late rheumatoid and psoriatic arthritis: comparison with a mathematical model. Arthritis Rheum. 2000;43:865–71.
5. Dhir V, Aggarwal A. Psoriatic arthritis: a critical review. Clin Rev Allergy Immunol. 2013;44:141–8.
6. McGonagle D. Enthesitis: an autoinflammatory lesion linking nail and joint involvement in psoriatic disease. J Eur Acad Dermatol Venereol. 2009;23 Suppl 1:9–13.
7. Zochling J, Smith EU. Seronegative spondyloarthritis. Best Pract Res Clin Rheumatol. 2010;24:747–56.
8. Joaquim AF, Appenzeller S. Cervical spine involvement in rheumatoid arthritis – a systematic review. Autoimmun Rev. 2014;13:1195–202.
9. Symmons DP, Silman AJ. Aspects of early arthritis. What determines the evolution of early undifferentiated arthritis and rheumatoid arthritis? An update from the Norfolk Arthritis Register. Arthritis Res Ther. 2006;8:214.
10. Emad Y, Anbar A, Abo-Elyoun I, El-Shaarawy N, Al-Hanafi H, Darwish H, et al. In palindromic rheumatism, hand joint involvement and positive anti-CCP antibodies predict RA development after 1 year of follow-up. Clin Rheumatol. 2014;33:791–7.
11. Scott DL, Steer S. The course of established rheumatoid arthritis. Best Pract Res Clin Rheumatol. 2007;21:943–67.
12. Young A, Koduri G. Extra-articular manifestations and complications of rheumatoid arthritis. Best Pract Res Clin Rheumatol. 2007;21:907–27.
13. Doyle TJ, Lee JS, Dellaripa PF, Lederer JA, Matteson EL, Fischer A, et al. A roadmap to promote clinical and translational research in rheumatoid arthritis-associated interstitial lung disease. Chest. 2014;145:454–63.
14. Sen D, Gonzalez-Mayda M, Brasington Jr RD. Cardiovascular disease in rheumatoid arthritis. Rheum Dis Clin North Am. 2014;40:27–49.
15. van der Horst-Bruinsma IE, Nurmohamed MT, Landewe RB. Comorbidities in patients with spondyloarthritis. Rheum Dis Clin North Am. 2012;38:523–38.

Chapter 4
Clinical and Laboratory Assessments

Abstract A number of clinical and laboratory methods have been developed to measure both the disease activity and severity of inflammatory arthritis patients. The most frequently used clinical measure to assess arthritis activity is joint counts (counting the number of swollen and tender joints, usually in 28 pre-specified joints). These are often combined with other clinical and laboratory measures in a composite score called the disease activity score on a 28-joint count (DAS28). Many measures of assessing inflammatory arthritis severity exist. In clinical practice the commonest methods include X-ray and ultrasound imaging, which capture joint damage and inflammation, and the health assessment questionnaire (HAQ), which provides information on function and disability. This chapter will provide a comprehensive overview of the methods used to assess the activity and severity of patients with an inflammatory arthritis.

Keywords Disease Outcomes • Disease Activity • Joint Counts • Radiography • Disability • Quality of Life

I.C. Scott et al., *Inflammatory Arthritis in Clinical Practice*,
DOI 10.1007/978-1-4471-6648-1_4,

Role of Assessments

The presence of an inflammatory arthritis is relatively easy to diagnose. The presence of painful, swollen joints is usually self-evident to both patients and clinicians. However, dividing patients into specific diagnostic groups can be challenging. Equally difficult is determining changes in the severity of arthritis over time. Clinical and laboratory assessments are vital to making informed decisions about diagnosis classification and disease severity.

Assessments used in patients with arthritis include joint counts, assessments of global health, patient self-assessments of disability and quality of life, laboratory assessments of disease activity and autoantibody status and imaging assessments of joint inflammation and joint damage [1]. Often a number of these various assessments are linked together to give composite scores of disease activity.

Clinical Assessments

Joint Counts

The characteristic features of inflamed joints comprise swelling and tenderness [2]. Joint swelling is soft tissue swelling detected along joint margins. When there is a synovial effusion, a joint is inevitably swollen. Effusions are not however mandatory features of a swollen joint. The most characteristic feature of a swollen joint is fluctuation, in which fluid can be displaced by pressure in two planes.

Bony swelling and joint deformities often complicate the counting of swollen joints. Neither of these indicates the presence of joint swelling, although they can be present when joints are swollen. In late disease it is often difficult to differentiate swollen from deformed inactive joints.

Joint tenderness is indicated by inducing pain in a joint at rest with pressure. Judging the correct amount of pressure to elicit tenderness depends on both the examiner and the patient. Generally sufficient pressure should be exerted by the examiner's thumb and index finger to cause 'whitening' of the examiner's nail bed; this equates with a pressure of approximately 4 kg/cm^2. In some joints, like the hip, tenderness is best identified through movement.

Many joints can be involved in inflammatory arthritis. Their size and distribution varies substantially, making it difficult to know how best to summate counts. A number of different joint counts have been devised. Initially developed counts assessed all 86 peripheral joints. For many years 66 joints were counted, including the joins in the feet. Currently joint counts usually assess 28 peripheral joints and exclude those in the feet.

When 28 joints are counted there are different assessments of swollen joints and tender joints. The joints assessed are shown in Fig. 4.1 and comprise:

- 10 proximal interphalangeal joints
- 10 metacarpophalangeal joints
- 2 wrist joints
- 2 shoulder joints
- 2 elbow joints
- 2 knee joints.

There are two limitations of using 28-joint counts. Firstly, they imply all joints are identical. However, joints like the knee are substantially larger than some of the interphalangeal joints. Although this can be addressed by correcting the count for the size of the joint involved, such corrections are rarely undertaken. Secondly, they ignore joints in the feet, and these can often be active when the hands are uninvolved. Nonetheless the 28-joint count is as effective as all other approaches.

There is no exact number of swollen or tender joints that mean arthritis is active. However, most experts suggest that 6 swollen and 6 tender joints indicate active disease and none or one swollen and tender joints represent low disease activity or remission.

FIGURE 4.1 Joints
assessed in 28 joint
counts

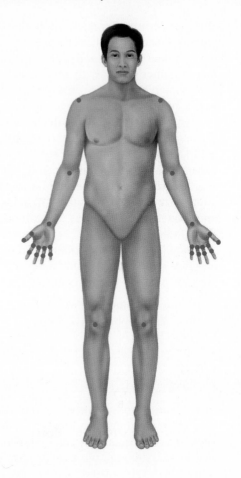

Examples of tender and swollen joint counts in 1,712
patients with RA attending our clinics are shown in
Fig. 4.2. Only a few patients have many active joints. Most
patients have no active joints or only one or two tender
and swollen joints. In addition the number of tender
joints is somewhat greater than the number of swollen
joints.

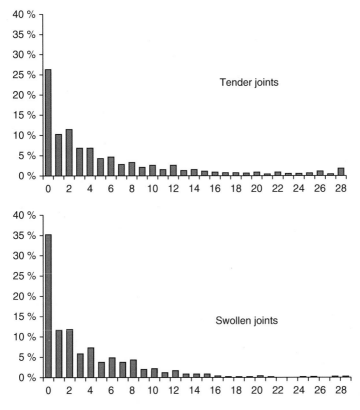

FIGURE 4.2 Joint counts in 1,712 patients with rheumatoid arthritis seen at King's College Hospital, London

Global Assessments

Global or overall assessments by patients and by clinicians are often used to assess disease activity. They are conventionally recorded using visual analogue scales (VAS). These score responses on 100 mm scales. Descriptive Likert scores have also been used; these group responses into distinct categories. Typically there are five categories which range from strongly

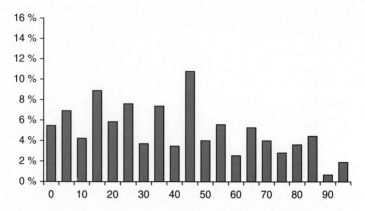

FIGURE 4.3 Patient global assessments in 1,712 patients with rheumatoid arthritis seen at King's College Hospital, London

agree to strongly disagree. High scores by patients and clinicians represent active arthritis.

One issue is which clinician should assess patients. Specialist rheumatologists, specialist nurses and allied health professionals, and a range of different healthcare professionals can all be involved. Their views are not entirely comparable. There is no correct answer and the range of assessments can be instructive and relevant.

The subjective nature of global assessments limits their overall value in determining disease activity. Some observers are optimistic while others are pessimistic. This makes comparisons between patients and observers less useful than changes over time within one individual's observations.

Examples of patient global assessments in 1,712 patients with RA attending our clinics are shown in Fig. 4.3. There is a wide range of different levels of response in patients. Unlike joint counts, which are distributed to the left side, there is a relatively even distribution of patient global responses across the whole range of possible scores. This indicates that patients' views of their arthritis are somewhat different from the objective assessments made by clinical assessors.

Pain Scores

Pain is usually considered to be a 'subjective' measure because its assessment is based on data obtained from the patient, which contrasts with 'objective' data from physical examination and laboratory tests [3]. However, quantitative estimations of levels of pain can only be obtained from patients and there is no alternative source.

There are a variety of ways of assessing pain. All of these are based on patient self-reported pain. The simplest approach, which is suitable for both research and routine practice, is to use a VAS. The standard VAS is a 10-cm scale bordered on each side. At the '0' mark, it says 'No pain at all', and at the '10' mark, 'Pain as bad as it could be'. Pain is then recorded as the length in millimetres from the zero mark on the scale.

An alternative is to use categories of pain. These provide five or more categories. For example none, minimal, moderate, severe and very severe. Such simple categorical scales are known as Likert scales. Both VAS and Likert scales provide similar information, but the Likert scales are less often used.

Pain is recorded within composite health status measures like the SF-36. There are also more complex pain scores that can be used in arthritis. An example is the McGill Pain Questionnaire. These are restricted to research studies.

There are several practical problems in using pain VAS scores. Firstly, they are better at measuring short term changes in pain. Patients have difficulties retaining any memory of pain severity over months or years. Secondly, they are influenced by the way patients complete VAS scores. Some patients use the full scale while others are more restricted and use only a small region of the scale. This makes it difficult to compare one patient's pain scores with another; the scores are better at defining changes in individual patients. Finally, some patients feel pain with a minimal stimulus compared to others. This is the concept of pain thresholds. Pain scores are usually high in patients with low pain thresholds and vice versa.

Functional Assessments

Function can be measured using "objective" measures of observed performance, but this approach has largely been abandoned in favour of assessments based on self-completed questionnaires that record patients' perception of their function.

The Health Assessment Questionnaire (HAQ) is the most widely used self-completed questionnaire to assess disability. It was developed over 30 years ago at Stanford. It focuses on self-reported, patient-oriented outcome measures [4].

HAQ assesses upper and lower limb function related to the degree of difficulty encountered in performing a number of specified daily living tasks. It assesses eight different domains of function. Each of these is scored on a range of zero to three. These indicate tasks can be undertaken without any difficulty (zero) or the patient is unable to do them (three). The highest score in each domain is used to calculate the overall HAQ score. The domains comprise dressing and grooming, arising, eating, walking, hygiene, reach, grip, and chores or activities

The scores from these eight domains are added to create a 0–24 point score which is then reduced to a 0–3 scale by dividing by eight. A HAQ score of zero 0 represents no disability. A score of 3 represents very severe disability and high dependency. HAQ scores can be measured in a range of different languages.

The reason for creating a 0–3 scale is historical. It allowed HAQ scores to be related to the initial functional score, which used a scale of I-IV grading for function; I was normal and IV completed disabled. A HAQ score of zero was linked to a functional grading of I and a score of 3 to a functional grading of IV. HAQ superseded the four-point functional score because it was better able to detect small changes in function.

HAQ is a very useful assessment but it has some limitations. One problem is that there are floor and ceiling effects. This means that low levels (floor) and high levels (ceiling) of disability are not recorded accurately by HAQ scores. This is a problem in applying HAQ to diverse groups of patients. In patients in the community with low levels of disability HAQ does not fully capture their problems. It also has limitations in assessing highly disabled patients from specialist centres with multiple problems.

Another specific problem in measuring disability is that HAQ scores are not linear. Although HAQ looks like a simple number line, it does not perform as one. A change from zero to one is not the same in terms of its impact on an individual patient as a change from 2 to 3.

A third limitation is that the change in HAQ scores that produce clinically noticeable changes from the perspective of individual patients is relatively high. Most experts believe a change in HAQ scores of 0.22–0.25 is required for patients to notice a difference in function. This means that the score is acting at the margin of detectable change as most drug treatments produce this level of change compared to placebo therapy.

A final problem is patients' perceptions of disability change as their arthritis progresses. In early arthritis HAQ scores can be high whilst in later disease they can be lower. The initial high HAQ scores in early arthritis improve when patients receive effective treatments. They then increase slowly as there is loss of muscle strength and a general increase in joint damage. But the increases are very slow and along the way patients change their perception of disability. In addition, with advancing age all people show some increase in disability due to the effects of aging.

Many other functional assessments have been used in arthritis. These include the Arthritis Impact Score and the Lee functional index. None of these have achieved the wide usage of HAQ scores.

Generic Health Status Measures

A number of generic health status measures are sometimes used in arthritis [5]. These include the SF-36, the Nottingham Health Profile and the EuroQol. The SF-36 and EuroQol are the dominant measures. Though they are rarely used in clinical practice, they have important research roles. Unlike disease specific assessments, they can be applied in all diseases and health states. They can therefore help compare the impact of arthritis with that of other medical disorders.

SF-36

The SF-36 is the dominant health state measure. It has been developed over 25 years and is available in almost all languages. It assesses health in 8 domains to give an overall health profile. Unlike most other measures zero represents poor health and 100, the upper end of each scale is perfect health. The SF-36 can be divided into two broad subscales assessing physical health and mental health. These are the physical summary scale and the mental summary scale.

The eight subscores assess physical function (2 scales), pain, vitality (broadly equivalent to fatigue), global health, social function and mental health (2 subscales).

Like HAQ there are problems with ceiling and floor affects and the SF-36 is relatively insensitive to measuring change in arthritis [6]. However, it provides a powerful picture of the overall impact of arthritis, which extends far beyond effects on physical function and pain alone. SF-36 scores in arthritis can be compared to scores for normal populations defined by age and sex and also by country.

EuroQol

The EuroQol, which is also known as EQ-5D, is a simpler measure that attempts to assess health status on a single line from zero (equivalent to death) to one (equivalent to complete health). It asks questions across a series of five domains. The questions are rather simple and the scoring is complex so that some health states score below zero, which is effectively worse than dead. The measurement properties of the EuroQol make it relatively unhelpful in arthritis. However, as it is often used in health economic studies and its overall importance in rheumatic diseases should not be underestimated.

Laboratory Assessments

Quantitative laboratory markers like the erythrocyte sedimentation rate (ESR) are useful for monitoring because they are a consequence of systemic disease. Qualitative markers like RF indicate prognosis and may have pathogenic relevance.

Acute Phase Response

Inflammation in the joints as elsewhere involves a systemic reaction as well as a local reaction. The systemic reaction is often termed the acute phase response. It can be measured in many different ways. However, the main tests are the erythrocyte sedimentation rate (ESR) and the C-reactive protein (CRP). Serum amyloid A protein tests are more sensitive but are rarely used due to technical limitations in the immunoassay method.

ESR and CRP levels are closely related to most clinical measures of disease activity [7]. In early arthritis they are mainly related to joint swelling. A persistently elevated acute phase response is associated with high rates of progressive joint damage. They provide more objective measures of disease activity than clinical assessments alone. The acute phase response occurs as a response to many different causes of inflammation. High levels of the ESR and CRP are therefore non-specific features in arthritis.

The ESR is the rate at which red blood cells precipitate in a period of 1 h when anti-coagulated blood is placed in an upright tube. The rate at which blood sediments is measured and reported in mm per hour (mm/h). The ESR reflects the balance between pro-sedimentation factors, especially

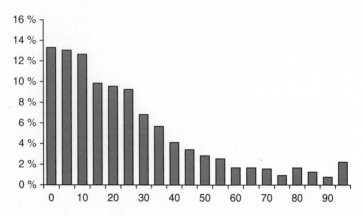

FIGURE 4.4 ESR levels in 1,712 patients with rheumatoid arthritis seen at King's College Hospital, London

fibrinogen, and factors resisting sedimentation, particularly small charge on the red blood cells. During inflammatory high levels of fibrinogen increases the rate of sedimentation. As the ESR is affected by many different proteins it is a very non-specific test. It is, however, often measured when evaluating the activity of inflammatory arthritis patients. Examples of ESR levels in 1,712 patients with RA attending our clinics are shown in Fig. 4.4. Over half the patients have raised ESR levels; some are very elevated at over 90 mm/h.

CRP is a single plasma protein. It was initially identified as a substance in the serum of patients with acute inflammation that reacted with the *C* polysaccharide of *pneumococcus*. This gave rise to its name. However, it is increased in all types of inflammation.

Although an elevated acute phase response is an excellent marker for disease activity, at presentation in over one third of patients with inflammatory arthritis both the ESR and CRP are normal. This is particularly true in AS patients with purely spinal involvement. In those patients in whom it is elevated, the acute phase response provides an excellent "flag" for the catabolic processes of arthritis. The aim of treatment is to return the elevated acute phase proteins towards normal.

Multi-biomarker Disease Activity (MBDA) Tests

An alternative to using single assays is the use of panels of different laboratory markers. An example of this is the Multi-Biomarker Disease Activity (MBDA) test [8]. This approach uses multiple biomarkers to assess disease activity levels. Starting with a large panel of possible protein biomarkers, the developers of this approach ended up with a panel of 12 biomarkers. They measure different biological pathways involved in RA pathogenesis. They can be broadly grouped into acute-phase response measures, hormones, growth factors, adhesion molecules, skeletal-related proteins, metallo-proteinases and cytokine related proteins.

An MBDA score is derived using an algorithm based on results in the 12 different biomarker levels. It divides patients into different levels of activity from active to remission. It is currently a commercially available assay, which is most widely used in North America. The extent to which it will be generally taken up is at present uncertain.

Rheumatoid Factor

These are antibodies directed against the Fc portion of immunoglobulin G (IgG). All classes of immunoglobulin can form RF. RF and IgG combine together as immune complexes. The immune disturbance of RA is influenced by these immune complexes.

Most patients with RA have RF in their synovial fluid and blood [9]. The exact frequency varies between centres. Overall 60–80 % of RA patients possess significantly elevated levels of RF. They are termed "seropositive" while those who are persistently RF-negative are termed "seronegative" patients. Measuring RF is an essential part of diagnosing RA, and RF tests are incorporated in all classification criteria for the disease.

The first RF tests used agglutination methods. This includes the classical Rose-Waaler tests based on sheep red cells and latex tests. These mainly detect IgM RF.

Newer solid phase techniques, particularly enzyme-linked immunosorbent assays (ELISA) can measure IgG and IgA RF isotypes. IgA RF, which is elevated in over half of RA patients, is potentially a good maker of disease severity and potential joint damage. However, research in this area has given conflicting results. Consequently measuring RF isotypes has not become part of routine practice.

RF is not specific for RA. It can be present in a wide variety of conditions in which there is disturbed immunity. Examples include connective tissue diseases, chronic inflammatory condition such as tuberculosis and are often seen in otherwise healthy people. Its frequency rises with age.

RF, especially in high titre in early disease, identifies patients with a poor prognosis. It is a good overall indicator of disease severity and is closely related to the development of erosive disease and extra-articular features such as nodules.

Antibodies to Citrullinated Protein Antigens

These antibodies have been measured in various forms since the 1960s. They were first described as antibodies to keratin and similar proteins in a range of cells, including buccal musosal cells and keratinised oesophageal cells in animal sections. They were variously termed anti-perinuclear factor, anti-keratin antibodies, and anti-filaggrin antibodies.

For over a decade all these antibodies have been known to target citrullinated proteins. Citrulline is a non-standard amino acid. It is formed from arginine by enzymic degradation. Citrullination occurs as part of the inflammatory reaction. A number of ELISA assays can detect antibodies to citrullinated proteins. The current second generation assays used cyclic epitopes carefully selected from libraries of citrullinated peptides to provide the most sensitive assays. The antibodies are variously known as antibodies to citrullinated protein antigens, which is shortened to ACPA, and Cyclic Citrullinated Peptide Antibodies, which is shortened to anti-CCP. ACPA has become the preferred term [10].

ACPAs are equally sensitive but more specific for RA than RF assays. Their sensitivity rates have been estimated at 60 %, which is similar to RF. However specificity rates are estimated at 96 %, compared to 86 % with RF.

There are several related autoantibodies, such as antibodies to vimentin. At present these are not used in routine practice. It is possible the range of autoantibodies tested will increase with time.

Both ACPA and RF may be present before the clinical onset of RA. In one study about half of 79 patients with RA had positive serology 5 years before the onset of their disease [11]. The presence of these antibodies can predict the development of RA in patients with an early undifferentiated arthritis. Additionally they predict more severe disease, with "antibody-positive RA" having more joint damage and fewer remissions compared with "antibody-negative RA".

Imaging

The commonly used imaging approaches are plain X-rays, ultrasound and MRI [12]. Other methods that are used less often include computerised tomography (CT), which has limited value in peripheral joints, and radio-isotope scans, which are now rarely used to diagnose or assess arthritis.

X-Rays in Rheumatoid Arthritis

X-rays in RA show many changes. These include soft tissue swelling, periarticular osteoporosis, loss of joint space, juxta-articular bony erosions, subchondral cysts, subluxation and ankylosis. Most changes are not specific and expert observers often disagree about their presence and extent. Erosions are the most diagnostic feature. Examples of erosions at the metacarpophalangeal and metatarsophalangeal joints in RA patients are shown in Fig. 4.5; these sites are classical areas for erosive damage in RA.

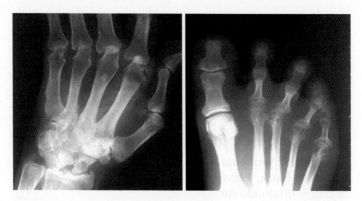

FIGURE 4.5 Erosive X-ray changes in the hands and feet in rheumatoid arthritis patients seen at King's College Hospital, London

The progression of X-ray changes provides an objective measure that is useful for both following the course of RA and assessing the long-term effects of treatment. Once the radiological cascade of damage starts, rapid progression is seen in the early years. In the later phases the rate of progressive damage tapers. Rapid X-ray progression indicates the need for more aggressive treatment especially at an early stage where it may be possible to avoid or abort subsequent major joint damage. The progression and increase of radiographic scores correlates with disease duration. The curve of radiographic progression ranges from linear in early stages, through an S-shape to flattening of the rate of progression at later stages.

There are many methods to quantify the amount and progression of x-ray damage. There are two widely used approaches. The Sharp method scores most of joints in the hand and wrist on a graded scale for erosions and narrowing. The Larsen method scores radiological appearances compared to a set of reference X-rays.

X-rays have several limitations as outcome measures and their place as one of the gold standards of RA outcome has been challenged. One problem is the frequency of floor and ceiling effects of the scoring system used (i.e. even though the highest score has been reached further deterioration can occur).

A second problem is that it can be difficult to determine if erosions have increased in size or if the position of the joint is slightly different from a previous radiograph. Finally, they may not directly reflect a patient's functional disability.

Ultrasound in Rheumatoid Arthritis

High-resolution ultrasound is better than clinical examination and conventional X-rays in diagnosing and assessing joint and bursal effusions and synovitis. It is the imaging modality of choice for tendon pathologies. It is also more sensitive at detecting erosions.

The main changes seen on ultrasound comprise:

- Effusions
- Synovial swelling indicating synovitis
- Tendonitis and tendon rupture
- Erosions

Doppler ultrasound, particularly power Doppler or colour Doppler imaging, allows an assessment of synovial vascularity. It can distinguish inflamed and non-vascular synovial swelling. The advantages of ultrasound are that it is relatively inexpensive, non-invasive and allows many joints to be assessed at any one time. It can be done in real time within the clinic and yields instant information. Its main disadvantage is its dependency on the skills of the operator and potential problems with reproducibility.

Ultrasound uses two approaches to evaluate joints. These are greyscale and power Doppler. Greyscale ultrasonography shows structures of the joints and surrounding tissues to be seen. Fluid and solid structures can be differentiated in their echotexture. Solid structures like are hyperechoic. Fluid appears anechoic. Doppler ultrasonography allows the blood flow to be visualized by the change in frequency of sound waves reflected by moving objects (the Doppler shift). It can slow velocity flow signals which suggest inflammation within joints and tendons. An example of these ultrasound approaches in an RA patient is given in Fig. 4.6. Marked

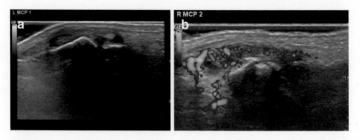

FIGURE 4.6 Ultrasound of a metacarpophalangeal joint demonstrating active synovitis in a rheumatoid arthritis patient seen at King's College Hospital, London. Panel (**a**) synovial hypertrophy on grey scale; Panel (**b**) synovial inflammation on power Doppler

power Doppler signal is seen indicating active synovitis at the metacarpophalangeal joint.

Magnetic Resonance Imaging in Rheumatoid Arthritis

MRI gives excellent images in arthritis and can show soft-tissue changes, cartilage changes, bony erosions and inflammatory change in the synovium. Gadolinium-based intravenous contrast agents are useful for defining the extent and severity of synovitis. MRI is the most sensitive approach for identifying destructive changes in early arthritis and for defining the benefits of early treatments. It remains more of a research investigation at present.

Imaging in Psoriatic Arthritis

Although the features are similar to RA, there is an asymmetric distribution, fewer joints are involved progression is less marked and bone proliferation is common. Specific changes include bony proliferation including periarticular and shaft periostitis, osteolysis with a "pencil in cup" deformity and acro-osteolysis and spur formation [13].

The main differences to RA include:

- Asymmetrical erosions in the wrists and metacarpopha-langeal joints
- Erosions of distal interphalangeal joints
- Erosive changes irregular due to periosteal bone formation
- Erosions progress to "pencil in cup deformity" with marked osteolysis

Imaging in Ankylosing Spondylitis and Reactive Arthritis

The main changes are in the spine and sacroiliac joints (which is a spinal problem rather than a form of inflammatory arthritis). Periarticular osteoporosis, loss of joint space and bone erosion are all seen in the peripheral joints [14]. Proliferation about sites of erosion is more characteristic of ankylosing spondylitis. In advanced disease periosteal reaction and proliferation at sites of tendon insertion are commonplace. A good example is the presence of exuberant plantar spurs.

Combined Measures

Core Data Set in Rheumatoid Arthritis

In RA no single measure is universally appropriate. The benefits of treatment are usually derived from a reduction in symptoms or slowing down the progression of the disease rather than achieving a cure. Until recently the outcome measures in both clinical trials and routine practice were chosen more by chance than design and there was no agreement on which, if any, measure was best. In the last few years a limited "core" set of preferred outcome measures has been defined by international consensus. These should be included in every clinical trial in RA and are suitable for routine practice. They comprise as follows:

- Number of swollen joints
- Number of tender joints
- Pain assessed by the patient
- Patient's global assessments of disease activity
- Assessor's global assessments of disease activity
- Laboratory evaluation (ESR, CRP, or equivalent)
- Self-administered functional assessment (e.g. Health Assessment Questionnaire)
- X-ray assessment for joint damage

Composite Disease Activity Indices: Disease Activity Score

There are many composite indices to assess RA [15]. The first to be widely used was the disease activity score (DAS). It was developed from a large prospective study in the Netherlands, which related the decision of rheumatologists to start or stop treatment to high and low levels of disease activity. By modeling clinical decisions a composite index was developed, which was termed DAS.

The original DAS used four measures: the Ritchie articular index, the swollen Joint Count based on 44 joints, the ESR and patients' general health assessment on a visual analogue scale. Subsequently, DAS was changed to assess fewer joints, using the 28 joint counts. The modified measure was termed the DAS28. It combines tender joint counts, swollen joint counts, the ESR and patients' global scores.

DAS28 is calculated using a complex formula:

$$0.56 * SqrtTJC28 + 0.28 * sqrtSJC28 + 0.70 * InESR + 0.014 * General Health$$

There have been further modifications of DAS including the development of a measure using CRP in place of ESR. All scores measure the same thing, though the numbers are slightly different.

DAS28 has become the leading European index. It is simple to use and is equally valid as more comprehensive articular indices, which can be time consuming to use in routine practice. DAS28 scores in rheumatoid arthritis fall into four categories, ranging from remission to high disease activity. These categories of DAS28 scores are as follows:

- Under 2.6: Remission
- 2.6–3.2: Low Disease Activity
- 3.3–5.0: Moderate Disease Activity
- 5.1 or more: High Disease Activity

Simplified Indices

As DAS28 requires complex calculations two simple indices have been developed. They are un-weighted and un-transformed. As a result they are easy to calculate. Most clinicians can calculate them in the clinic.

The first of these is the simplified disease activity index (SDAI). This uses five variables, including the CRP level. The second is the clinical disease activity index (CDAI), which has no laboratory variables. These simplified indices are closely related to DAS28. They have different numeric cut-off points. They are less often used in routine clinical practice.

The components of these simplified indices are as follows:

- SDAI: number of swollen joints (our of 28) + number of tender joints (our of 28) + patient's global assessment (on 10 cm visual analogue scale) + physician's global assessment (on 10 cm visual analogue scale) + CRP (mg/dL)
- CDAI = number of swollen joints (our of 28) + number of tender joints (our of 28) + patient's global assessment (on 10 cm visual analogue scale) + physician's global assessment (on 10 cm visual analogue scale)

American College of Rheumatology (ACR) Response Criteria

These were developed in 1995 to simply the assessment of response in clinical trials. They use components of the core data set and involve improvements in both swollen and tender joint counts and three out of: patient global assessment, physician global assessment, pain, ESR and a functional measure such as HAQ. Improvements can be at 20, 50 or 70 % levels (termed ACR-20 to ACR-70 responses). Although ACR response criteria are widely used in trials, they are not relevant in clinical practice.

Other Forms of Arthritis

Although DAS28 and ACR response criteria can be used in other forms of arthritis, they are less useful when only a few joints are involved.

In PsA there are Psoriatic Arthritis Response Criteria (PsARC) [16]. These comprise the following:

- patient global self-assessment
- physician global assessment
- tender joint score
- swollen joint score

It does not include an assessment of psoriasis. A response is defined as an improvement in at least two of the four measures, one of which has to be the joint tenderness or swelling score, with no worsening in any of the four measures.

In AS there are a number of different measures to assess its overall severity. The most widely accepted is the Bath Ankylosing Spondylitis Disease Activity Index (BASDAI). This consists of 10 cm visual analogue scales that evaluate six questions related to the major symptoms of the disorder. These comprise:

- Fatigue
- Spinal pain

- Joint pain and swelling
- Areas of localized tenderness (*enthesitis* or inflammation of tendons and ligaments)
- Morning stiffness duration
- Morning stiffness severity

To give each symptom equal weighting, the average of the two scores relating to morning stiffness is taken. The resulting 0–50 score is divided by 5 to give a final zero to ten BASDAI score. Scores of 4 or greater suggest suboptimal control of disease and the need for additional treatment.

Outcomes

Rheumatoid Arthritis

The outcome of treated RA includes assessments of joint damage, disability, mortality and the costs of the disease. Each of these types of outcome has different implications for patients, healthcare providers and clinicians treating the disease. They are inter-related at a global level in that on average patients who show marked radiological damage also have the most disability, higher mortality and greater costs. However, there are marked individual variations and many patients have considerable radiological damage, but little disability and vice versa some cases have considerable disability and little damage [17].

In early RA the key change is the development of juxta-articular erosions. In the first few years of RA, between 50 and 75 % of patients will develop one or more erosions in their hands and wrists. Those patients who have no erosions by 3 years are unlikely to develop them later in the disease. In late disease the main problem is end-stage joint damage. In early disease less than 5 % of joints are totally damaged. After 20 years of RA about 20 % of joints are completely damaged, and many of these will need surgical replacement.

During the course of RA, between 5 and 20 years of disease there is a steady progression of joint damage. Longitudinal studies show that in early disease on average patients have less than 20 % of maximal possible damage. By 20 years this has increased to about 50 % of maximum possible damage, an increase of 1–3 % per year. Damage to large joints is a major cause of disability in later disease.

Average HAQ scores in groups of patients increase with disease duration. After 5–7 years of RA average HAQ score are about 0.8 (27 % maximum possible disability). These increase in a linear manner by 1–3 % per year so that by 18–20 years they are in the region of 1.11 (37 % maximum possible disability). There is a different pattern of HAQ scores in the first 5 years of rheumatoid arthritis in which there is a "J-shaped" curve. HAQ scores fall initially, when patients with active disease receive effective treatment. They then increase in a stepwise manner.

There are more deaths in RA patients from all causes than in people of similar age and sex without arthritis. Standardised mortality ratios (SMR), which allow comparisons across different populations, show RA patients have SMRs for all cause of death between 1.1 and 3.0 relative to the general population. In keeping with the general causes of death in Europe and North America, heart disease is the commonest cause of death in RA patients. The way in which RA patients are chosen for mortality studies influences the results. Hospital based RA patients have higher SMRs than community cases; suggesting disease severity is an important indicator of premature death.

Cardiovascular diseases such as myocardial infarctions and strokes cause 40–50 % of mortality in the general population and in patients with RA. Both of these show an increase in RA compared to normal controls. Cardiac deaths are most likely in patients who are seropositive for rheumatoid factor. Other factors may also be involved, including steroid treatment, diabetes mellitus and hypertension.

Overall cancer deaths are not increased in rheumatoid arthritis. However, there is one exception. RA patients have a markedly, and possibly time-limited, increased risk for malignant lymphomas. There is little to suggest these excess results from inherited or environmental risk factors in malignant lymphomas. Instead, lymphomas complicating RA appear to be a direct consequence of the inflammation or its treatment. At the same time the number of RA patients who develop lymphomas is small, as the disease is relatively uncommon.

Psoriatic Arthritis

Patients with PsA have reduced quality of life and limited function compared with patients with psoriasis alone or healthy controls [18]. The overall impact of the disease is similar to that of RA. The severity of PsA is shown by the gradual increase in joint damage that occurs over its course and the increased mortality. The excess of death is in the region of 60 % with a SMR of about 1.6. The causes of death are similar to those in the general population, with cardiovascular causes being the commonest. The risk for premature death is increased with active and severe disease, the presence of erosive disease, and a high ESR when first seen.

Ankylosing Spondylitis

Although there is less information about the long-term outcomes of AS, they appear equally severe to those in RA. Patients have reduced function, impaired quality of life and some increase in mortality. The data for AS represents the impact of less intensive treatments and it may be improving with more active management using biologics.

References

1. Anderson J, Caplan L, Yazdany J, Robbins ML, Neogi T, Michaud K, et al. Rheumatoid arthritis disease activity measures: American College of Rheumatology recommendations for use in clinical practice. Arthritis Care Res. 2012;64:640–7.

2. Scott IC, Scott DL. Joint counts in inflammatory arthritis. Clin Exp Rheumatol. 2014;32:S-7-12.

3. Englbrecht M, Tarner IH, van der Heijde DM, Manger B, Bombardier C, Muller-Ladner U. Measuring pain and efficacy of pain treatment in inflammatory arthritis: a systematic literature review. J Rheumatol Suppl. 2012;90:3-10.

4. Bruce B, Fries JF. The Stanford Health Assessment Questionnaire: dimensions and practical applications. Health Qual Life Outcomes. 2003;1:20.

5. Coons SJ, Rao S, Keininger DL, Hays RD. A comparative review of generic quality-of-life instruments. Pharmacoeconomics. 2000;17:13-35.

6. Matcham F, Scott IC, Rayner L, Hotopf M, Kingsley GH, Norton S, et al. The impact of rheumatoid arthritis on quality-of-life assessed using the SF-36: a systematic review and meta-analysis. Semin Arthritis Rheum. 2014;44:123-30.

7. Pincus T, Sokka T. Laboratory tests to assess patients with rheumatoid arthritis: advantages and limitations. Rheum Dis Clin North Am. 2009;35:731-4.

8. Centola M, Cavet G, Shen Y, Ramanujan S, Knowlton N, Swan KA, et al. Development of a multi-biomarker disease activity test for rheumatoid arthritis. PLoS One. 2013;8:e60635.

9. Shmerling RH, Delbanco TL. The rheumatoid factor: an analysis of clinical utility. Am J Med. 1991;91:528-34.

10. Suwannalai P, Trouw LA, Toes RE, Huizinga TW. Anti-citrullinated protein antibodies (ACPA) in early rheumatoid arthritis. Mod Rheumatol. 2012;22:15-20.

11. Nielen MMJ, van Schaardenburg D, Reesink HW, van de Stadt RJ, van der Horst-Bruinsma IE, de Koning MHMT, et al. Specific autoantibodies precede the symptoms of rheumatoid arthritis: a study of serial measurements in blood donors. Arthritis Rheum. 2004;50:380-6.

12. McQueen FM. Imaging in early rheumatoid arthritis. Best Pract Res Clin Rheumatol. 2013;27:499-522.

13. Bakewell CJ, Olivieri I, Aydin SZ, Dejaco C, Ikeda K, Gutierrez M, et al. Ultrasound and magnetic resonance imaging in the evaluation of psoriatic dactylitis: status and perspectives. J Rheumatol. 2013;40:1951-7.

14. Ostergaard M, Poggenborg RP, Axelsen MB, Pedersen SJ. Magnetic resonance imaging in spondyloarthritis–how to quantify findings and measure response. Best Pract Res Clin Rheumatol. 2010;24:637-57.

15. Anderson JK, Zimmerman L, Caplan L, Michaud K. Measures of rheumatoid arthritis disease activity: Patient (PtGA) and Provider (PrGA) Global Assessment of Disease Activity, Disease Activity Score (DAS) and Disease Activity Score with 28-Joint Counts (DAS28), Simplified Disease Activity Index (SDAI), Clinical Disease Activity Index (CDAI), Patient Activity Score (PAS) and Patient Activity Score-II (PASII), Routine Assessment of Patient Index Data (RAPID), Rheumatoid Arthritis Disease Activity Index (RADAI) and Rheumatoid Arthritis Disease Activity Index-5 (RADAI-5), Chronic Arthritis Systemic Index (CASI), Patient-Based Disease Activity Score With ESR (PDAS1) and Patient-Based Disease Activity Score without ESR (PDAS2), and Mean Overall Index for Rheumatoid Arthritis (MOI-RA). Arthritis Care Res. 2011;63 Suppl 11:S14–36.

16. Mease PJ. Measures of psoriatic arthritis: Tender and Swollen Joint Assessment, Psoriasis Area and Severity Index (PASI), Nail Psoriasis Severity Index (NAPSI), Modified Nail Psoriasis Severity Index (mNAPSI), Mander/Newcastle Enthesitis Index (MEI), Leeds Enthesitis Index (LEI), Spondyloarthritis Research Consortium of Canada (SPARCC), Maastricht Ankylosing Spondylitis Enthesis Score (MASES), Leeds Dactylitis Index (LDI), Patient Global for Psoriatic Arthritis, Dermatology Life Quality Index (DLQI), Psoriatic Arthritis Quality of Life (PsAQOL), Functional Assessment of Chronic Illness Therapy-Fatigue (FACIT-F), Psoriatic Arthritis Response Criteria (PsARC), Psoriatic Arthritis Joint Activity Index (PsAJAI), Disease Activity in Psoriatic Arthritis (DAPSA), and Composite Psoriatic Disease Activity Index (CPDAI). Arthritis Care Res. 2011;63 Suppl 11:S64–85.

17. Kingsley G, Scott IC, Scott DL. Quality of life and the outcome of established rheumatoid arthritis. Best Pract Res Clin Rheumatol. 2011;25:585–606.

18. Gladman DD, Antoni C, Mease P, Clegg DO, Nash P. Psoriatic arthritis: epidemiology, clinical features, course, and outcome. Ann Rheum Dis. 2005;64 Suppl 2:ii14–7.

Chapter 5
Symptomatic Drug Treatment

Abstract   As pain is the main symptom that inflammatory arthritis patients report, analgesics are a major focus of their management. Simple analgesics such as paracetamol and Non-Steroidal Anti-Inflammatory Drugs (NSAIDs) are commonly used. Both have risks when used long-term. A particular concern with long-term NSAID use is an increased risk of cardiovascular and gastrointestinal events such as myocardial infarction and gastro-oesophageal bleeding. This chapter will provide a broad overview of symptomatic drug treatments in inflammatory arthritis patients. It will focus on the different classes of available treatments, their relative merits and disadvantages, alongside their use in the different forms of inflammatory arthritis.

Keywords   Analgesics • Paracetamol • NSAIDs • Side-effects

Introduction

Pain is the dominant symptom in arthritis. It is present from the earliest stages of synovitis and persists throughout the course of the disease. In early inflammatory arthritis pain is predominantly related to the activity of the synovitis. In late disease it is influenced by the development of joint damage and failure.

I.C. Scott et al., *Inflammatory Arthritis in Clinical Practice*,
DOI 10.1007/978-1-4471-6648-1_5,
© Springer-Verlag London 2015

Pain in arthritis overlaps with chronic pain generally, which is a major medical problem. Nearly half the adult population report chronic pain. It is particularly prevalent in the elderly and is also associated with poverty, being retired and being unable to work. Arthritis is the commonest cause of pain in the community.

The impact of poorly controlled pain cannot be overestimated in inflammatory arthritis. Almost all patients with inflammatory arthritis report pain is a major health problem. Pain has close links with psychological symptoms including depression and anxiety. It is also closely related to disability and impaired health status.

There are several ways to control pain. The first and most important is to give symptomatic drug treatment with analgesics or anti-inflammatory drugs. The second is to control the underlying inflammatory disease process. The third is to replace damaged joints, which is only relevant in late disease. Finally non-specific measures such as exercise therapy or treating co-existent depression also reduce pain, and the benefits of anti-depressants may extend beyond merely treating depression into a direct effect on pain itself.

Other important symptoms in arthritis stem from joint inflammation. Pain is accompanied by joint tenderness, swelling and stiffness, together with morning stiffness. Symptomatic treatment with anti-inflammatory drugs improves stiffness and tenderness and to some extent will reduce joint swelling. The effect of symptomatic treatment on joint tenderness and swelling is less than that of disease modifying treatments.

Simple Analgesics

Simple analgesics should be used in all patients with inflammatory arthritis as an adjunct to non-steroidal anti-inflammatory drugs (NSAID) and DMARD therapy. The available drugs include paracetamol, co-proxamol and tramadol (Table 5.1). Although there is some evidence from clinical trials that analgesics reduce pain in RA, the amount of data

TABLE 5.1 Commonly used analgesics

Simple	Compound
Paracetamol	Co-codamol (paracetamol/codeine)
Codeine	Co-dydramol (paracetamol/ dihydrocodeine)
Dihydrocodeine	
Tramadol	
Buprenorphine	

is very limited. Most trials of these drugs were carried out more than 20 years ago and by current standards did not study enough patients and did not last long enough. However, almost all rheumatologists recommend using them. At the same time, only a very small proportion of patients with RA and other inflammatory arthropathies will have their disease controlled by analgesics alone.

Paracetamol

Paracetamol is the dominant analgesic. It is effective with a single dose of 1,000 mg paracetamol providing more than 50 % pain relief over 4–6 h in moderate or severe pain compared with placebo. Its analgesic effects are comparable to those of conventional NSAIDS, there are virtually no groups of people who should not take it, interactions with other treatments are not a problem, at the recommended dosage there are virtually no side-effects, it is well tolerated by patients with peptic ulcers.

Interestingly despite being used for many years the mechanism of action of paracetamol is not well understood. It may be centrally active, producing analgesia by elevation of the pain threshold by inhibiting prostaglandin synthetase in the hypothalamus. At therapeutic dosages it does not inhibit prostaglandin synthetase in peripheral tissues, and consequently has no anti-inflammatory activity.

Although paracetamol has been used to control symptoms in inflammatory arthritis for many years, the evidence supporting its efficacy remains weak [1]. The weakness of this evidence is, however, partly related to the historic nature of the drug. The evidence base for many long-standing drugs is weak because the need for strong evidence when they were introduced was minimal.

One limitation with paracetamol is that it is relatively ineffective, patients need to take 6–8 tablets daily to achieve any analgesic benefit, and most patients prefer to take NSAIDs. Patients' perspectives highlight the limitations of paracetamol. Only a minority of patients find it is effective and the majority prefer NSAIDs for symptom control.

Historically the safety of paracetamol has been emphasised. However, there are concerns about its potential toxicity with therapeutic doses. These include:

- liver injury, especially in patients with underlying liver disease, malnutrition and chronic alcohol use
- renal disease, with evidence of reduced renal function in patients who have taken paracetamol
- hypertension, which has been identified as a possible risk in large observational studies.

Opioids

These are widely used to control pain. In arthritis weak opioids (codeine, dextropropoxyphene and tramadol) are often used, whist strong ones (morphine and its derivates) are avoided. Although these drugs are effective in chronic non-cancer pain, many patients stop taking them due to side effects. These reactions include nausea, constipation and drowsiness.

The reasons that strong opiates like as morphine are virtually never used in treating inflammatory arthritis are complex. It is usually thought that their addictive nature makes their over value more disadvantageous than beneficial. However, this view is based on custom and practice rather than any rigorous scientific testing. A small minority of patients do benefit from them. There is reasonable evidence opioids are effective in improving symptoms in inflammatory arthritis, particularly patient-reported pain levels, although adverse events such as nausea are not uncommon (Fig. 5.1) [2].

Tramadol

Tramadol is effective in relieving moderate to moderately severe pain. It is a weak synthetic opioid that also has serotonin-releasing and noradrenaline reuptake inhibitory properties. It is used to treat moderate to severe pain in arthritis. Tramadol causes less constipation than conventional opiates. Dependence is not a clinically relevant problem. To be fully effective tramadol needs to be given at a dose of 50–100 mg every 4–6 h. A slow release formulation can be useful if night pain is a particular problem. Its most frequent adverse effects include headache, dizziness and somnolence.

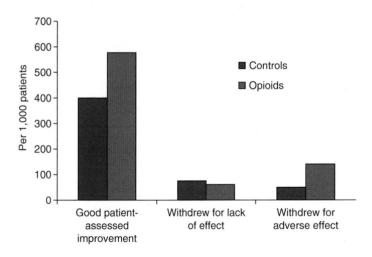

FIGURE 5.1 Efficacy and toxicity of opioids in rheumatoid arthritis (From systematic review by Whittle et al., figure adapted using data reported by Whittle et al. [2])

The sleepiness caused by tramadol often precludes its use in patients who need to be mentally alert in the day. Tramadol is closely regulated and in the United Kingdom it is now classified as a schedule three controlled drug.

Buprenorphine

Buprenorphine is now available as a transdermal preparation for treating the pain of arthritis. It is an opioid analgesic. The patches have reservoirs of buprenorphine which is slowly absorbed into the blood. Patches need to be changed weekly to deliver continuous pain relief. The use of transdermal treatment reduces some of the adverse effects of opiates such as constipation and nausea. It also provides more continuous efficacy.

Codeine and Dihydrocodeine

These weak opioids have centrally mediated effects. They are effective after 20–30 min and last for about 4 h. Dihydrocodeine has about twice the potency of codeine. They show a ceiling effect for analgesia and higher doses give progressively more adverse effects, particularly nausea and vomiting. These adverse effects outweigh any additional analgesic effect.

Compound Analgesics

Patients can combine paracetamol with a weak opiate as single agents or in combination tablets. Co-proxamol, which is the combination of paracetamol with dextropropoxyphene (an agent that is rarely used alone), was historically popular with clinicians. There was no obvious reason for this and the drug has been withdrawn from general use. Currently available combinations comprise paracetamol with codeine (co-codamol) or dihydrocodeine (co-dydramol). These compound drugs have the same effects and adverse reactions as individual drugs.

Non-steroidal Anti-inflammatory Drugs (NSAIDs)

NSAIDs are a diverse group of drugs with a name that was introduced to distinguish them from glucocorticoids and the non-narcotic analgesics. Overall NSAIDs are one of the most frequently used group of drugs. Their benefits must be set against significant risks from gastrointestinal and renal toxicity, which cause a substantial number of deaths each year.

Mechanism of Action and Cox I/Cox II Effects

Inflammation involves many locally produced chemical mediators. These include prostaglandins, leukotrienes, complement-derived products, and products of activated leukocytes, platelets and mast cells.

The central and most important effect of NSAIDs is inhibiting cyclo-oxygenase (COX). COX has been presumed to be the major target of NSAIDs for many years influencing their analgesic and anti-inflammatory capacities. It was originally purified in the 1970s. By 1990 it was realised the enzyme had two isoforms, termed Cox I and Cox II [3]. The first isoform – COX-1 – is responsible for the production of "housekeeping" prostaglandins critical for normal renal function, gastric mucosal integrity and vascular haemostasis. By contrast COX-2 is an inducible enzyme. It is upregulated in macrophages, monocytes and other inflammatory cells by various stimuli including interleukin-1 and other cytokines. NSAIDs can be classified according to their relative effects on Cox I and Cox II. The risk of GI adverse effects seems to be reduced with increasing Cox II selectivity. However, other factors are involved, as some NSAIDs that are relatively Cox II selective are known to be associated with a higher incidence of GI adverse events.

Several types of assays assess the Cox-II selectivity. In vitro human whole blood assay is an accepted and reproducible standard. However it may not truly reflect the Cox inhibition in target tissues like the gastric mucosa. Recent assays use human target cells such as gastric mucosal cells and synovio-cytes. There are wide variations in ratios reported by using different assay techniques. Results from in vitro testing are no more than a general guide to the relative in vivo selectivity of different drugs.

NSAIDs have many other actions including uncoupling oxidative phosphorylation, inhibiting lysosomal enzyme release, inhibiting complement activation, antagonising the generation of activity of kinins, and inhibiting free radicals. None of these mechanisms can completely explain the actions of NSAIDs

Classification of NSAIDs

NSAIDs differ from each other and can therefore be classi-fied not only by their relative COX-1/COX-2 inhibition but also by their chemical class and their plasma half-life. They are mainly organic acids with low pKa values. These low pKa values may facilitate penetration of inflamed tissue, where pHs are often low. The more acidic drugs usually have shorter half-lives. There is marked individual variation in response to NSAIDs, though the causes of such variations are not known. Unfortunately this variability makes it difficult to predict how a patient will respond to NSAID treatment. NSAIDs are often produced in slow-release or sustained-release prepara-tions. These can allow once-daily dosing, and may reduce gastrointestinal side effects.

All NSAIDs exhibit anti-inflammatory properties and are often the first treatment given to patients with inflammatory arthritis. Their efficacy is readily shown in comparison to pla-cebo within 2 weeks in patients with active RA. Virtually all of the NSAIDs relieve pain when used in doses substantially lower than those required to demonstrate suppression of inflammation. The analgesic action of NSAIDs is generally considered to be peripheral, as opposed to the central effect of narcotics. There is some evidence of a possible blockade of pain transmission or perception of painful stimuli in the central nervous system and spinal cord by selective COX-2 inhibitors.

Conventional NSAIDs

Although many NSAIDs have been developed, in clinical practice most specialists use only a few drugs (Table 5.2). The earliest NSAIDs have either been withdrawn, in the case of phenylbutazone, or are only used infrequently, as in the case of indomethacin. This includes drugs that can be given between once and three times daily. Giving NSAIDs frequently provides greater flexibility in getting the best dose for an individual patient. At the same time it also means taking many more tablets at relatively frequent intervals. Giving an NSAID once daily is often more convenient, but this is offset by greater relative toxicity. The risks of toxicity with conventional NSAIDs can be minimised by giving the lowest dose compatible with symptom relief, and by reducing or stopping treatment when patients have achieved a good response to disease modifying drugs.

In choosing between different conventional NSAIDs, it is important to realise that systematic reviews have found no major differences in efficacy between the currently available NSAIDs over a range of doses. However, they have found differences in adverse reactions. Many of the early conventional NSAIDs have been withdrawn due to concerns about adverse events, or they are rarely used because of their high relative toxicity.

Cox-2 Drugs (COXIBs)

The discovery of the two COX isoenzymes was a significant advance. COX-2 was considered to provide anti-inflammatory action and pain relief, as seen with conventional NSAIDs, but

TABLE 5.2 Commonly used non-steroidal anti-inflammatory drugs

Drug	Suggested dose	Advantages	Limitations
Conventional NSAIDs			
Diclofenac	75 mg slow release bd	Rapid onset of action and relatively good efficacy	Concerns about liver toxicity
Ibuprofen	600 mg tds	Well known and widely used with short half-life giving great flexibility of use	Requires frequent dosing
Naproxen	500 mg bd	Effective when used twice daily	Standard NSAID with no major drawbacks though no evidence it has more long-term safety
COXIBs			
Celecoxib	200 mg bd	Reduced gastric toxicity	Some unresolved concerns about cardiac adverse events
Etoricoxib	90 mg daily	Reduced gastric toxicity and once daily dosing	Fluid retention makes it unsuitable for patients with cardiac failure

without the toxicity associated with COX-1 inhibition. This concept led to the development of a new class of drugs that specifically inhibit COX-2 while sparing COX-1. Although a number of COXIBs have been developed only two are used to any great extent. These are celecoxib and etoricoxib. Other COXIBs were all withdrawn due to potential adverse reaction risks.

There is a substantial body of evidence from large trials, some of which are of long duration that show Coxibs like celecoxib are effective in RA. They improve both tender joint counts and pain scores in RA patients (Fig. 5.2) [4]. These drugs are more effective than placebo and equally effective as maximum daily doses of standard NSAIDs (such as diclofenac and naproxen).

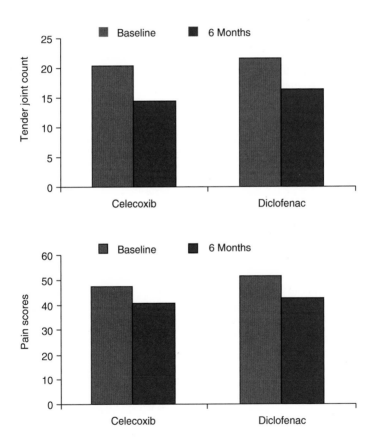

FIGURE 5.2 Efficacy of NSAIDs in rheumatoid arthritis: a double-blind randomised comparison of celecoxib versus diclofenac (Figure adapted using data reported by Emery et al. [4])

Adverse Reactions to NSAIDs

This is the major limiting factor to using NSAIDs. As a class NSAIDs are probably the commonest group of drugs for causing adverse events (Table 5.3). The risks increase markedly with age and NSAIDs must be used carefully in the elderly. Minor adverse effects such as dyspepsia and headache are commonplace. Central nervous system side-effects, such as drowsiness and confusion, are often underestimated. Hematologic side-effects are very unusual. NSAIDs can also exacerbate asthma and cause rashes, though these are usually mild.

Prostaglandins regulate kidney function, especially intrarenal perfusion. As a consequence NSAIDs inevitably carry

TABLE 5.3 Adverse reactions to NSAIDs

Area	Type of adverse reaction
Gastrointestinal	Dyspepsia
	Peptic ulceration
	Small bowel ulcers and enteropathy
Renal	Acute and chronic renal failure
	Interstitial nephritis
Cardiovascular	Exacerbation of cardiac failure
	Exacerbation of hypertension
Hepatic	Elevated transaminases
	Hepatic failure (rare)
Central nervous system	Headache
	Drowsiness
	Confusion
Haematological	Thrombocytopenia
	Haemolytic anaemia

a risk of adversely effecting renal function. These renal side effects are dose-dependent and occur in a small but consistent proportion of patients. Common problems comprise peripheral oedema, hypertension, and reduced effects of diuretics and anti-hypertensive drugs. When renal blood flow is reduced, for example by cardiac failure or diuretic use, the added inhibition of prostaglandin synthesis by NSAIDs further impairs blood flow, and this can cause overt renal failure. This problem is particularly likely in the elderly. Other renal problems seen occasionally include acute renal failure, hyperkalaemia, and interstitial nephritis and papillary necrosis.

Gastrointestinal Adverse Effects

These side effects are the main problem with NSAIDs. The range of adverse effects includes dyspepsia, gastric erosions, peptic ulceration, bleeding, perforation, haematemesis or melaena, small bowel inflammation, occult blood loss and anaemia.

Between 10 and 20 out of every 1,000 RA patients taking NSAIDs for 1 year will have serious gastrointestinal complications. The mortality risks attributable to NSAID-related GI adverse effects are four times that for those not using NSAIDs. There is some evidence that gastro-intestinal mortality from NSAIDs is similar in its extent to other major causes of death such as melanoma and leukaemia. The most serious problems are perforations, ulcers and bleeds. There is some evidence that the risk of GI adverse events differs across NSAIDs (Fig. 5.3) [5].

Many patients who have serious gastro-intestinal complications do not have prior dyspepsia. In the absence of warning signs there is no way to ascertain if a patient is on the point of developing serious problems. Therefore if NSAID use is unavoidable, some protective strategy is needed, particularly in those patients at greatest risk. There are several potential options.

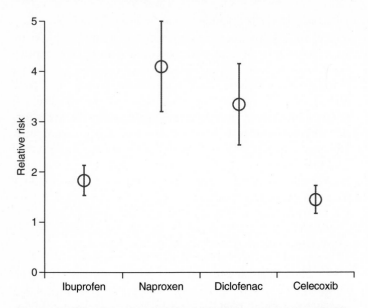

FIGURE 5.3 The risk of gastrointestinal adverse events stratified by NSAID type (From systematic review by Castellsague et al., figure adapted using data reported by Castellsague et al. [5])

One choice is to co-prescribe proton pump inhibitors, such as omeprazole. This is effective and acceptable to patients. H2-receptor antagonists also help, but are less effective than proton pump inhibitors. A third choice is to co-prescribe prostaglandin analogues, such as misoprostol. This is also effective, but causes added side effects such as diarrhoea and is less well tolerated than proton pump inhibitors. The final option is to use a safer NSAID – one of the newer COX-2 drugs.

Although COXIBs increase the incidence of gastrointestinal adverse events compared to placebo, the magnitude is substantially less than with standard NSAID therapy. They reduce the incidence of gastric erosions on endoscopy compared to standard NSAIDs. However, the value of this finding as a surrogate for peptic ulceration and other major gastrointestinal adverse effects in routine clinical practice is uncertain. Many experts also recommend combining proton pump inhibitors with COXIBs to maximise gastrointestinal safety.

The key evidence focuses on their effect on peptic ulcerations, perforations and bleeds. These have been studied in a number of large trials involving several thousand patients. The balance of evidence is that these drugs reduce serious upper gastro-intestinal adverse events to the same level as that seen with placebo treatment and substantially below that with conventional NSAIDs.

These are broadly similar to those seen with conventional NSAIDs. Patients still have renal, central nervous system and other effects. However, there is also no evidence of any increases in other adverse effects, so the overall benefit for patients taking these drugs remains significant.

Cardiovascular Adverse Effects

There have been concerns that NSAIDs in general and COXIBs in particular increase the risk of heart attacks and strokes. The data about cardiovascular risks with NSAIDs overall is controversial and incomplete. Some trials and some observational studies have found more cardiac problems; other trials have not done so [6]. Overall the risk of myocardial infarction on conventional NSAIDs appears small, although the risk may vary depending on the type of conventional NSAID used (Fig. 5.4) [7].

One COXIB – rofecoxib –shows an increased risk in most circumstances [7]. It was consequently withdrawn. Other COXIBs and conventional NSAIDs do not show an increased risk in most situations. However, they need to be given with caution. It is generally recommended that the lowest dose for the shortest period of time is a sensible policy. Patients at risk of cardiac disease should not receive NSAIDs, and in particular should avoid COXIBs. As well as cardiac infarctions some drugs, including rofecoxib, have an increased risk of fluid retention and can cause an increased propensity to cardiac failure.

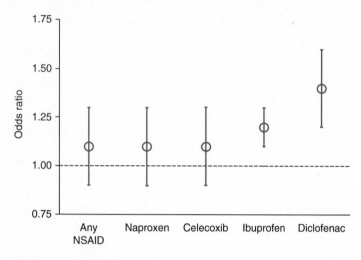

FIGURE 5.4 The risk of cardiovascular adverse events stratified by NSAID type (From systematic review by Scott et al., figure adapted using data reported by Scott et al. [7])

On the other hand, any potential cardiac risks of COXIBs are offset by a reduction in risk of serious gastrointestinal ulcers and other major upper gastrointestinal adverse events.

Use in Specific Forms of Arthritis

Rheumatoid Arthritis

Historically NSAIDs were considered first line treatment in RA. However, this classical approach is now considered inappropriate and patients need to start disease modifying drugs as soon as possible. This issue is discussed in detail in the following chapters.

Currently analgesics and NSAIDs are used to provide additional symptomatic control in RA, when pain and morning stiffness are dominant symptoms which are not controlled by disease modifying therapy alone [8, 9].

A few patients with mild disease can manage on NSAIDs and analgesics alone. However, in the majority of patients they are used intermittently to gain improved control of symptoms. They are best avoided for long-term treatment.

In some patients taking disease modifying drugs, particularly methotrexate, there can be interactions with NSAIDs. Caution is needed in these patients. Elderly patients, and those with multiple comorbidities, are most likely to have adverse effects with NSAIDs and their use should be minimised in these patients.

Psoriatic Arthritis and Seronegative Spondyloarthritis

The situation is somewhat different in PsA and there is a greater emphasis on the early use of NSAIDs in these patients [10, 11]. The balance of expert opinion is unanimous in recommending NSAIDs as first-line treatment for most patients with psoriatic arthritis, though there is a general realisation that the data supporting their value is limited. NSAIDs are effective in reducing joint symptoms in patients with psoriatic arthritis. They have no benefits on skin lesions.

When using NSAIDs risks of gastrointestinal and cardiovascular adverse events need to be considered. Not all patients with signs and symptoms of psoriatic arthritis need NSAID treatment. Some patients respond well to analgesics alone. Others may not need any symptomatic therapy. As with all patients the lowest dose and the shortest treatment duration possible is appropriate when using NSAIDs in these patients.

Ankylosing Spondylitis

NSAIDs are highly effective in AS and are also recommended for non-radiographic axial spondyloarthritis [12]. They rapidly improve inflammatory back pain and stiffness.

However, concerns about their long-term safety and their adverse effects lead to NSAIDs being stopped in many patients. The risks associated with NSAIDs make many clinicians reluctant to prescribe continuous NSAID therapy. Some experts favour this approach, and it might result in less radiographic progression of spinal AS. However, this remains a controversial issue. Nevertheless the balance of evidence suggests trying to control symptoms in all AS patients using NSAIDs. Analgesics can sometimes provide some additional benefit.

References

1. Hazlewood G, van der Heijde DM, Bombardier C. Paracetamol for the management of pain in inflammatory arthritis: a systematic literature review. J Rheumatol Suppl. 2012;90:11–6.
2. Whittle SL, Richards BL, Husni E, Buchbinder R. Opioid therapy for treating rheumatoid arthritis pain. Cochrane Database Syst Rev. 2011;(11):CD003113.
3. Vane JR, Botting RM. Anti-inflammatory drugs and their mechanism of action. Inflamm Res. 1998;47 Suppl 2:S78–87.
4. Emery P, Zeidler H, Kvien TK, Guslandi M, Naudin R, Stead H, et al. Celecoxib versus diclofenac in long-term management of rheumatoid arthritis: randomised double-blind comparison. Lancet. 1999;354:2106–11.
5. Castellsague J, Riera-Guardia N, Calingaert B, Varas-Lorenzo C, Fourrier-Reglat A, Nicotra F, et al. Individual NSAIDs and upper gastrointestinal complications: a systematic review and meta-analysis of observational studies (the SOS project). Drug Saf. 2012;35:1127–46.
6. Trelle S, Reichenbach S, Wandel S, Hildebrand P, Tschannen B, Villiger PM, et al. Cardiovascular safety of non-steroidal anti-inflammatory drugs: network meta-analysis. BMJ. 2011;342:c7086.
7. Scott PA, Kingsley GH, Smith CM, Choy EH, Scott DL. Non-steroidal anti-inflammatory drugs and myocardial infarctions: comparative systematic review of evidence from observational studies and randomised controlled trials. Ann Rheum Dis. 2007;66:1296–304.

8. Wienecke T, Gotzsche PC. Paracetamol versus nonsteroidal anti-inflammatory drugs for rheumatoid arthritis. Cochrane Database Syst Rev. 2004;(1):CD003789.
9. Chen YF, Jobanputra P, Barton P, Bryan S, Fry-Smith A, Harris G, et al. Cyclooxygenase-2 selective non-steroidal anti-inflammatory drugs (etodolac, meloxicam, celecoxib, rofecoxib, etoricoxib, valdecoxib and lumiracoxib) for osteoarthritis and rheumatoid arthritis: a systematic review and economic evaluation. Health Technol Assess. 2008;12:1–278.
10. Nash P, Clegg DO. Psoriatic arthritis therapy: NSAIDs and traditional DMARDs. Ann Rheum Dis. 2005;64 Suppl 2:ii74–77.
11. Gossec L, Smolen JS, Gaujoux-Viala C, Ash Z, Marzo-Ortega H, van der Heijde D, et al. European League Against Rheumatism recommendations for the management of psoriatic arthritis with pharmacological therapies. Ann Rheum Dis. 2012;71:4–12.
12. Guellec D, Nocturne G, Tatar Z, Pham T, Sellam J, Cantagrel A, et al. Should non-steroidal anti-inflammatory drugs be used continuously in ankylosing spondylitis? Joint Bone Spine. 2014;81:308–12.

Chapter 6
Disease-Modifying Anti-Rheumatic Drugs

Abstract DMARDs are a diverse range of drugs. They form a single group because they both improve symptoms and modify the course of the disease. They form the cornerstone of inflammatory arthritis management. A range of DMARDs exist. Methotrexate is most commonly used in clinical practice, followed by sulfasalazine and hydroxychloroquine. All DMARDs have potential adverse events and require monitoring, often with blood tests. Historically patients were treated with a single DMARD at a time (termed DMARD monotherapy). There has been a recent shift towards starting more than one DMARD at the same time (termed DMARD combination therapy) in patients with RA. This chapter will provide an overview of the different available DMARDs, their mechanisms of action, risks and benefits alongside the evidence base supporting their use.

Keywords DMARD • Methotrexate • Sulfasalazine • Hydroxychloroquine • Efficacy • Side-Effects

Background

DMARDs are a diverse range of drugs. They form a single group because they both improve symptoms and also, to a greater or lesser extent, modify the course of the disease. This

TABLE 6.1 The range of Disease-Modifying Anti-Rheumatic Drugs (DMARDs) used

Frequency of use	DMARD		
Commonly used	Methotrexate	Leflunomide	Sulfasalazine
Infrequently used	Hydroxychloroquine	Injectable gold	Azathioprine
Rarely used	Ciclosporin	Auranofin	Cyclophosphamide

means they reduce the progression of erosive joint damage and decrease disability [1].

Ideally DMARDs would result in remission. However, there is little evidence that they generally achieve this goal. Their failure to do so led to the abandonment of an earlier term – "remission inducing drugs". Another collective term that has fallen out of use is "slow-acting anti-rheumatic drugs" [2]; this fell out of favour because in some patients these drugs may have relatively rapid onsets of action.

Currently Used Conventional DMARDs

Many drugs have some features of DMARDs, but only a few have been accepted into clinical practice. The use of DMARDs varies with a small number being particularly favoured. The current situation is summarised in Table 6.1. At present methotrexate is the dominant DMARD. Over 80 % of patients with rheumatoid arthritis treated with DMARDs who are seen in most specialist units are receiving methotrexate. Only sulfasalazine and leflunomide are also used to any appreciable extent in addition to methotrexate.

The use of DMARDs broadly follows the strength of evidence about their efficacy. The efficacy of DMARDs involves:

- Less joint inflammation with fewer swollen joints and falls in ESR and C-reactive protein
- Decreased progression of joint damage, particularly erosive damage
- Improved levels of disability and quality of life

The harms, or adverse events, related to DMARDs include:

- Common problems to most DMARDs like low white cell or platelet counts
- Unique toxicities with specific DMARDs, such as ocular toxicity with hydroxychloroquine.

A systematic review comparing trials of the main DMARDs concluded that methotrexate, sulfasalazine and leflunomide all showed similar efficacy and toxicity [3]. The main conclusions are shown in Table 6.2. One problem in these comparisons is that the trials involve one fixed dose against another fixed dose and in practice treatment is targeted at individual patients. Another problem in that older studies used doses of methotrexate that are currently considered to be suboptimal. However, for practical purposes the evidence suggests these three treatments are similar.

Starting DMARDs

In patients with definite rheumatoid arthritis DMARDs are started as soon as the diagnosis has been made. The evidence in favour of early DMARDs, though incomplete, is compelling. Most experts recommend starting with methotrexate.

Monitoring DMARDs

The risk of blood and hepatic toxicity means that most DMARDs require monthly blood monitoring tests. This practice began because it was possible to predict patients at risk of marrow toxicity with gold injections by prospective monitoring; this approach substantially improved safety risks. With modern treatment the risks are less clear cut and the benefits of monitoring are more questionable. However, in some patients adverse events involving the blood and liver can be detected on monitoring and such reactions carry substantial risks for patients. Consequently monitoring has become part of the standard approach to DMARD treatment [4].

TABLE 6.2 Comparison of efficacy and harms for different DMARD monotherapies

Comparison	Leflunomide vs. methotrexate	Leflunomide vs. sulfasalazine	Sulfasalazine vs. methotrexate
Efficacy	Similar improvements in joint inflammation and erosive damage	Greater improvements in joint inflammation for leflunomide	Similar improvements in joint inflammation, function and radiographic responses
	Greater improvement in functional status and health-related quality of life for leflunomide	Greater improvement in functional for leflunomide	
	Similar work productivity outcomes	Similar radiographic responses	
Harms	No obvious major differences in adverse events and discontinuation rates	No obvious major differences in adverse events and discontinuation rates	No obvious major differences in adverse events
			More patients received methotrexate than sulfasalazine

Table adapted using data reported by Donahue et al. [3]

Stopping DMARDs

DMARDs are stopped for toxicity and for loss of effect. Often these overlap. In patients who have entered remission or a state of low activity the benefit of continuing DMARDs is often questioned. The evidence suggests that stopping treatment in such patients often results in a disease flare; consequently it is not generally recommended [5].

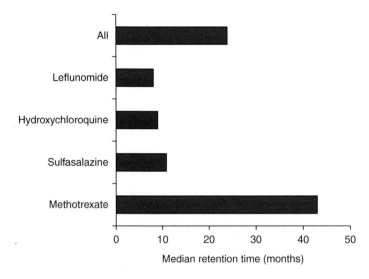

F<small>IGURE</small> 6.<small>I</small>   Retention rates for DMARDs in patients with rheumatoid arthritis (Figure adapted using data reported by Agarwal et al. [6])

The frequency of stopping DMARD monotherapies is high. Almost half of patients initiating DMARDs discontinue treatment over the next 2–3 years. Retention rates differ across DMARDs, with patients remaining on methotrexate longer than other DMARDs (Fig. 6.1) [6]. This finding has been confirmed in many different observational studies. Such low retention rates make it particularly crucial to consider carefully the benefits and risks of discontinuing DMARDs in patients in whom therapy is controlling RA and is not causing adverse effects.

Early and Late Disease

DMARD use is comparable in all stages of inflammatory arthritis. Patients who need DMARDs in early disease are equally likely to continue using them in later stages of the disease.

Intensive Treatment

Historically DMARDs were given singly – as DMARD monotherapy – but there has been a shift in practice over the last 2 years to using then in combination with each other. There are two ways of giving combination therapy:

- Step-down: starting combinations together and then stopping one or more DMARDs
- Step-up: starting one DMARD and then adding another if needed.

In addition combinations can involve two DMARDs, DMARDs and steroids, and DMARDs and biologics.

Ideally patients with the worst prognosis would be identified rapidly and then given intensive treatment to control their arthritis as soon as possible. However, this has proved problematic to do as at present it is difficult to identify patients with poor prognoses with sufficient accuracy to justify a policy of starting intensive DMARD combinations in specific groups of patients.

Treat to Target

The concept of "treat to target" builds on intensive management approaches in rheumatoid arthritis [7]. It sets a goal of reducing disease activity to very low levels or remission. With modern treatments this appears increasingly realistic. It should reduce long-term structural damage and improve quality of life. Treat to target involves setting a clear end point, which in this case is the target of remission, and establishing a specific treatment algorithm, which simplifies the many complex treatment sequences available to treat arthritis. However, there are some complexities. The definition of treat to target varies and a range of different data is used to justify its benefits. Some patients are reluctant to receive more intensive treatment due to concern over adverse effects. Finally, the evidence that remission is generally achievable in active rheumatoid arthritis is incomplete no matter how patients are treated.

Seronegative Arthritis

Seronegative rheumatoid arthritis responds similarly to seropositive disease. Patients with other forms of inflammatory arthritis such as psoriatic arthritis and reactive arthritis are treated in the same way as patients with rheumatoid arthritis. The evidence for using DMARDs in seronegative spondyloarthritis, particularly psoriatic arthritis, is weaker than that for rheumatoid arthritis. However, the evidence that DMARDs have different effects in any form of inflammatory arthritis is incomplete. Most rheumatologists consider they provide comparable results [8], though some experts are unconvinced about the role of methotrexate in psoriatic arthritis. One important point is that DMARDs do not appear to improve either the spinal disease or enthesopathy of seronegative spondyloarthritis [9].

Changes in Clinical Trials

Reduction in Joint Counts and Acute Phase Proteins

When patients are treated with DMARDs there are falls in their tender and swollen joint counts over 3–6 months (Fig. 6.2). After 6 months the joint counts stabilise and they do not fall further. Although there is a small improvement with placebo, there are larger falls with active DMARDs. Whether or not the effect of placebo is due to a specific response or is an example of "regression to the mean" is uncertain. Unfortunately some residual disease activity exists. The pattern of change is similar with other assessments of disease activity, including swollen joint counts and acute phase measures like the ESR.

After 6 months the reductions in clinical responses are maintained as long as patients remain on treatment [11]. This is shown for 1 and 2 years in Fig. 6.3. Overall the pattern of improvements is broadly similar with methotrexate,

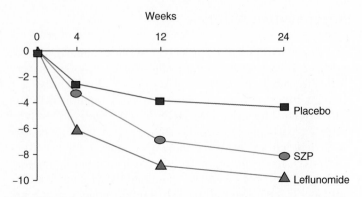

FIGURE 6.2 Falls in tender joint counts with placebo, sulfasalazine and leflunomide (Figure adapted using data reported by Smolen et al. [10])

leflunomide and sulfasalazine [10, 12]. There is no need to prefer one DMARD over another on the basis of clinical responses.

American College of Rheumatology Responses (ACR)

Effective DMARDs result in greater ACR20 and ACR50 responses over 6–12 months than placebo treatment. This is shown in Fig. 6.4 using the largest available trial data with DMARDs – the leflunomide Phase III trials – that involved the key three DMARDs and placebo treatment [13].

Improved Disability

DMARDs improve disability over 12 months or longer, especially in those patients who remain on treatment. This is seen with all major DMARDs. Health Assessment Questionnaire scores decreased by about one third with effective DMARD therapy and remained thereafter at this lower average level.

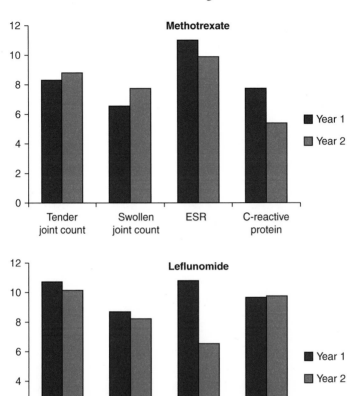

FIGURE 6.3 Falls in joint counts and acute phase reactants with methotrexate and leflunomide treatment (Figure adapted using data reported by Cohen et al. [11])

Radiological Damage

The evidence the different DMARDs reduce the progression of erosive damage is complex and not all studies give similar results. There are many ways of assessing damage and the

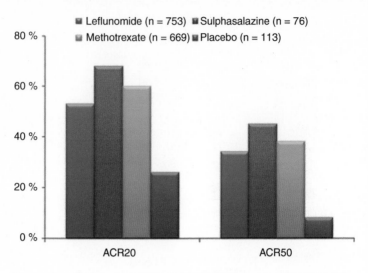

FIGURE 6.4 Changes in ACR20 and ACR50 responses with DMARDs (Figure adapted using data reported by Scott and Strand [13])

differences between them are complicated. A simple approach is shown in Fig. 6.5, which compares erosive progression with and without DMARDs in different trials [14]. One complexity is that fewer patients now show marked erosive progression during the course of their rheumatoid arthritis. This means that the rate of progression was more marked in earlier trials and the impact of DMARDs seemed larger.

Methotrexate

Background

Methotrexate has become the main DMARD. Although it is an elderly drug, which has been used for over 50 years, its rise to prominence in inflammatory arthritis is more recent. The balance of its efficacy, safety, ease of administration and patient acceptability has made it a key treatment option. It is now considered to be the "anchor drug" in treating

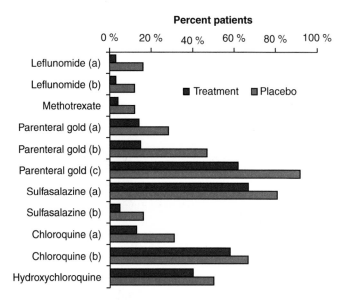

FIGURE 6.5 The chance of erosive progression with and without DMARDs (a, b and c refer to different studies of each DMARD; Figure adapted using data reported by Jones et al. [14])

inflammatory arthritis, and that this role may have been enhanced by its positive interaction with biologic treatments [15].

Methotrexate is an anti-metabolite; it inhibits folate metabolism, and was first used to treat cancer. In arthritis it used at low doses; at such doses it does not kill cells and exerts its effects on joint inflammation by other mechanisms. It affects adenosine metabolism, leucocyte accumulation and angiogenesis.

Clinical Use and Efficacy

Low-dose methotrexate in arthritis is given weekly. It is usually given by mouth but can be given by subcutaneous or intramuscular injections. Patient acceptability and adverse reactions determine which route is used. Methotrexate is strongly bound to plasma proteins; there is a theoretical risk of free methotrexate levels increasing because of displacement

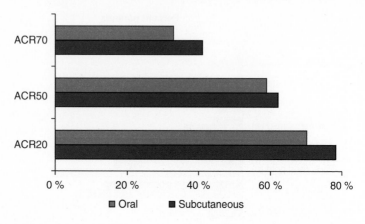

FIGURE 6.6 Six-month trial of oral and subcutaneous methotrexate (Figure adapted using data reported by Braun et al. [16])

from albumin by highly bound drugs like non-steroidal anti-inflammatory drugs, but this is not a practical problem.

Oral or parenteral (subcutaneous) methotrexate is usually started at doses between 7.5 and 10 mg/week. The dose is incrementally increased to target dose of 15–20 mg/week. This target dose has gradually increased over the years. Some experts recommend going up to 25 mg/week. If patients have difficulty tolerating higher doses the amount of methotrexate given can be restricted below 15 mg/week.

There is some evidence that subcutaneous methotrexate is more effective than oral treatment (Fig. 6.6) [16]. Therefore in patients in whom oral methotrexate gives incomplete responses some rheumatologists recommend converting to subcutaneous methotrexate improves efficacy.

Methotrexate is conventionally given with low dose folic acid, which reduces the risk of adverse reactions, particularly hepatic toxicity. It also reduces other gastrointestinal adverse effects. The optimal dose schedule is uncertain, though 5 mg weekly appears adequate. This level of folic acid supplementation has no more than a modest impact on efficacy.

A particular concern with methotrexate is ensuring patients do not inadvertently take the wrong dose. There are reports of patients taking methotrexate daily rather than weekly and also of patients receiving 10 mg tablets rather than 2.5 mg tablets. When prescribing methotrexate it is essential to ensure the dose is correct.

Adverse Reactions

Adverse events are common with methotrexate, though most events are minor and can usually be managed without stopping therapy. Some of the main problems are as follows:

- Gastrointestinal problems: these are dominant and include anorexia, nausea, vomiting and diarrhoea.
- Stomatitis: including erythema, painful ulcers and erosions
- Alopecia: this is frequent and causes particular concern in women.
- Other skin reactions: including urticaria, and cutaneous vasculitis.
- Central Nervous System problems: including headaches, drowsiness and ataxia
- General problems: examples include fever, fatigue and myalgias.
- Infections, including opportunistic infections with organisms like Pneumocystis carinii, fungal infections and localised or disseminated herpes zoster sometimes occur.

There are also a number of serious side effects including:

(a) Bone marrow toxicity: mild to moderate leucopenia, which responds to withdrawal of the drug. More severe bone marrow suppression may be treated with leucovorin or recombinant colony-stimulating factors.
(b) Liver toxicity: mild transaminase elevations are common but serious hepatotoxicity leading to fibrosis or cirrhosis is rare.
(c) Pulmonary interstitial disease: this can develop suddenly and may progress to fibrosis. It is sometimes fatal. It often occurs early in therapy. The development of a cough is often a warning feature. Patients need to have a plain chest x-ray before starting treatment.

Accelerated nodulosis, with small nodules on the fingers or elbows, occurs occasionally. The nodules are indistinguishable from other rheumatoid nodules. Some experts stop methotrexate and others suggest an additional drug like hydroxychloroquine.

Methotrexate is teratogenic and should not be given in pregnant women. Women taking methotrexate who may become pregnant need reliable methods of birth control. A 6 month delay after stopping methotrexate is recommended for women who wish to conceive. Breast-feeding is not recommended while taking methotrexate as the drug may enter the mother's milk.

Methotrexate may lower sperm counts in men; these normalise after it is stopped. It is conventional to recommend that males discontinue methotrexate for up to 6 months prior to attempting conception.

Leflunomide

Background

Leflunomide is the only new DMARD to have been introduced in the last two decades. It was developed as an immunosuppressant and acts as a pyrimidine synthesis inhibitor with consequential anti-proliferative activity. Leflunomide is a prodrug and is rapidly converted in the gastrointestinal tract and plasma to its active metabolite, a malononitrilamide, which is responsible for its activity in vivo.

The active metabolite of leflunomide has a range of effects, which include:

- Inhibiting pyrimidine synthesis: inhibits dihydroorotate dehydrogenase
- Inhibiting nuclear factor kappa-B activation
- Reducing cell-cell contact
- Reducing bone marrow cell proliferation
- Inhibiting synovial nitric oxide production

The effect on pyrimidine synthesis is mediated by the inhibition of dihydroorotate dehydrogenase, the rate-limiting step in the de novo synthesis of pyrimidines. Unlike other cells, activated lymphocytes expand their pyrimidine pool eightfold during proliferation. Thus the inhibition of dihydroorotate dehydrogenase prevents lymphocytes from accumulating sufficient pyrimidines to support DNA synthesis and has a consequent immunomodulatory effect. This is thought to be the main effect.

Peak levels of the active metabolite are seen 6–12 h after oral dosing. As the active metabolite has a long half-life, in the region of 2 weeks, loading doses of 100 mg for 3 days were used in the initial clinical studies to facilitate the rapid attainment of steady-state levels of the active metabolite. In the absence of a loading dose steady-state plasma concentrations require about 2 months of dosing.

Clinical Use and Efficacy

Rheumatologists have three different ways of starting leflunomide. Historically a loading dose was used of 100 mg daily for 3 days. This increased plasma levels rapidly and ensured a rapid onset of action. However, it may give higher risks of adverse events. An alternative is to start with the main dosage level of 20 mg daily and accept a slower onset of action with a reduced level of adverse events. In some patients where there are concerns about adverse reactions a lower starting dose of 10 mg is sometimes used. There is limited objective evidence supporting this more conservative approach.

Adverse Events

The profile of side effects with leflunomide is broadly similar to those seen with methotrexate. The main specific adverse reactions seen with leflunomide comprise:

- Gastrointestinal reactions, particularly diarrhoea are often seen; omitting the loading dose reduces the frequency and severity of diarrhoea.

- Hypertension is seen some cases, though it can be difficult to differentiate the effects of non-steroidal anti-inflammatory drugs from leflunomide in raising the blood pressure.
- Occasional patients report weight loss with leflunomide, though its relationship to therapy is uncertain.

As with other DMARDs there is also a small increased risk of infections, reflecting its role as an immunosuppressive agent. Haematological problems are sometimes seen and a few patients have developed low white cell counts or low platelet count; in these circumstances treatment needs to be stopped. Lung problems including interstitial lung disease have been seen with leflunomide; they are uncommon. Skin problems are often seen and may need treatment to be stopped.

A major cause of concern with leflunomide is liver damage. Transient increases in liver enzymes are commonplace, and usually need no more than careful observation. If the levels rise by more than three times normal treatment should be stopped. A few patients have developed cirrhosis or liver failure whilst taking leflunomide, though there is debate about causality. Caution is needed in patients with prior liver disease and those with significant alcohol intakes. To detect liver problems early patients need regular monitoring of liver function and also blood counts.

Leflunomide is a teratogenic DMARD, and should not be given to women who are at risk of pregnancy. Given the long half-life of the drug, it needs to be stopped for many months prior to conception, and some authorities recommend a 2-year period. Caution is also needed in men who wish to conceive.

There is a washout procedure for patients with severe side effects or in men or women considering conception. This involves giving cholestryamine or activated powdered charcoal for 1 or 2 weeks.

Sulfasalazine

Sulfasalazine combines an anti-inflammatory agent (5-aminosalicylic acid) with a sulfonamide antibiotic (sulfa-pyridine), which if often thought to be the active component.

There is extensive metabolism of sulfasalazine and its two constituents after the drug is taken. Its mechanism of action is unknown. However, there is experimental evidence that it inhibits T cells, B cells and cytokine production.

Sulfasalazine is given orally with a target dose is 2–3 g daily. To minimise upper gastrointestinal side effects such as nausea treatment is initiated at 500 mg daily rising slowly to 2 or 3 g. It is usually given in an enteric coated formulation, which also helps to minimise adverse effects.

Sulphasalazine causes may adverse effects in addition to gastrointestinal disturbances and these include:

- Haematological problems such as leucopenia, neutropenia, agranulocytosis and thrombocytopenia.
- Hypersensitivity reactions such as rashes, Stevens-Johnson Syndrome, exfoliative dermatitis, urticaria, photosensitisation, anaphylaxis, fever, lymphadenopathy and periorbital oedema
- Central nervous system problems such as vertigo and tinnitus
- Hepatic dysfunction, which is usually mild but can be severe.
- Oligospermia, which is reversible on discontinuance

It requires monitoring for blood and liver toxicity in the early stages. One especial concern is allergic neutropenia that occurs in both early and late treatment and is difficult to predict.

One specific advantage with sulfasalazine is that it can be used in pregnant women. Long-term clinical usage and experimental studies have failed to show any teratogenic hazards. Although caution is needed in breast feeding mothers, the amounts of drug present in the milk is not generally thought to present a risk to healthy infants.

Other DMARDs

Injectable Gold

Gold salts are the oldest DMARD and are also the most toxic. They take months before showing evidence of efficacy. Gold is usually given as gold sodium thiomalate, though gold sodium thioglucose can also be given.

The mechanisms by which gold work have been investigated for many years, but little is known. As the use of gold resulted from serendipity rather than design, there was no prior hypothesis about how it works. As its use predated the modern era by the time its effects could be reliably investigated there was little interest in evaluating them. In addition, injectable gold is a complex compound, and contains many constituents formed after manufacture.

Injectable gold is by weekly intramuscular injections (50 mg) for 20 weeks and then reduced to monthly. Based empirically on clinical experience, the following schedule is recommended: Initial "test doses" of 10 mg are given to minimize the risk of toxicity.

Adverse events are common with gold and often severe. These include post injection reactions, rashes, stomatitis and pruritus. Less common but more serious adverse reactions are the nephrotic syndrome, low white cell counts, thrombocytopenia, bone marrow aplasia, interstitial lung disease and peripheral neuropathies.

Hydroxychloroquine

This anti-malarial drug was used in rheumatology to treat systemic lupus erythematosus. Subsequent placebo-controlled trials confirmed its efficacy in rheumatoid arthritis. It is thought to be most useful in mild early disease. It is usually given at a dose of 400 mg/day. It is less effective than methotrexate or sulfasalazine. It has little effect on erosive damage.

Common adverse effects include rash, abdominal cramps and diarrhoea. Its main toxicity is the rare but highly unpleasant complication of retinopathy. Some form of retinal screening is recommended for patients starting hydroxychloroquine. Patients at higher risk of retinopathy, who are over 60 years of age, have over 5 years' treatment or use doses greater than 6.5 mg/kg/day, need regular review, with annual ophthalmological examination.

Ciclosporin

Ciclosporin is an immunosuppressant that is widely used in organ transplantation. It was used in inflammatory arthritis because of its immunosuppressive properties and effects on T-cell function. Although it is effective its use is limited by toxicity, which is dose dependent. Its adverse effects, particularly nephrotoxicity and hypertension, mean its long-term use is problematic. Though the decline in renal function seen in some patients taking ciclosporin is reversed when therapy is discontinued, this is a major limitation. Ciclosporin is usually confined to use in refractory RA when no other obvious therapeutic options are available.

Azathioprine

Azathioprine is also used because of its systemic immunosuppressive effects. It is a pro-drug of 6-mercaptopurine. Although it is effective; the results in trials are inconsistent. There is little evidence it affects erosive damage.

A particular concern is the risk of serious haematological toxicity. A relative decrease in the activity of the enzyme thiopurine methyltransferase is a risk factor for bone marrow suppression. Genotyping patients to identify those most at risk might prevent such adverse events. Azathioprine is mainly used in refractory disease when patients have failed other agents.

Minor DMARDs

Oral gold, penicillamine and cyclophosphamide are rarely used to treat inflammatory arthritis. Oral gold has limited efficacy and the other drugs have excessive toxicity. They are used in occasional patients in whom other options are limited.

Combining DMARDs

Rationale

As many patients fail to respond to conventional DMARD monotherapy there has been considerable interest in combining one or more DMARDs.

The arguments that have been used to justify combination therapy include the following:

- monotherapy is inadequate
- low doses of combined DMARDs improve toxicity and efficacy ratios
- using DMARDs sequentially deprives patients of residual benefits of the 'failed' drug
- sequential use of inadequate monotherapy means patients in the early critical phase of their disease are not well controlled.

Until recently there were concerns that combination DMARD therapy offered limited benefits over conventional monotherapy. However perspective has now changed and there is wide support for combination DMARDs [17].

Effective Combinations

1. Methotrexate, Hydroxychloroquine And Sulfasalazine: there is extensive evidence that this combination is both more effective than its component DMARDs and also less toxic. This is probably because the doses of each individual DMARD are minimised. Longer-term follow-up shows the benefits of treatment persist for 3 years. Combining any two of these three drugs, such as methotrexate and sulfasalazine, also has some benefits though these are less marked.
2. Methotrexate and Leflunomide: there is considerable evidence that combining leflunomide in patients with an incomplete response to methotrexate improves disease

activity without excessive adverse events. There have been concerns that this combination may give rise to excessive liver toxicity. Care is therefore needed when using it and careful monitoring of liver function is advisable.

3. Leflunomide and Sulfasalazine: there is some evidence this combination is moderately effective and safe.

4. Methotrexate and Ciclosporin: several studies show methotrexate can be combined with ciclosporin. Although problems of toxicity with ciclosporin remain, as its dose can be lowered these problems are minimised.

5. Methotrexate and Gold: there is some evidence this combination is effective and safe.

6. Leflunomide and Ciclosporin: there is limited evidence this combination is effective and safe.

Ineffective Combinations

Not all DMARD combinations are useful. With some there is limited efficacy or excessive toxicity. Combinations involving penicillamine appear ineffective. There is also evidence that combining gold injections with hydroxychloroquine has limited benefit and excessive toxicity.

Intensive Treatments in Early Disease

In early inflammatory arthritis combining two DMARDs with steroids, particularly an initially high dose that is reduced rapidly over a few months, is an attractive option in early disease. It was first described in a Dutch trial named the COBRA study, and is often termed the COBRA regimen [18]. The DMARDs involved can be methotrexate and sulfasalazine or methotrexate and ciclosporin. There is no evidence of excessive toxicity. A particular feature of this approach is the reduction in the progression of erosive damage, which can be marked. Some experts replace the high dose, short-term steroid regimen with either intermittent intra-muscular steroids or with lower doses of oral steroids.

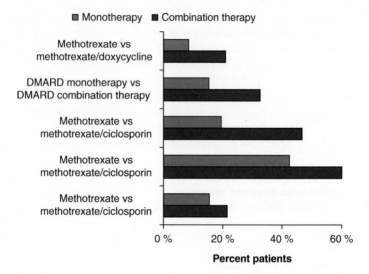

FIGURE 6.7 The impact of combination DMARDs on ACR70 responses, supporting the use of combination therapy (Figure adapted using data reported by Ma et al. [19])

Overall Effectiveness of Combinations

There is compelling evidence that combinations are preferable to monotherapy. An example of these benefits is shown by the impact on ACR70 responses from a review by Ma et al. (Fig. 6.7) [19]. However, not all experts reach identical conclusions using the same data and trials. This is because there are many different ways to combine DMARDs and the conclusions are influenced by whether all trials of all combinations are considered or if each type of combination is viewed separately.

Seronegative Spondyloarthritis

There is limited data and very few trials of using combination DMARDs in patients with psoriatic arthritis and other forms of seronegative arthritis. Some experts consider this is an appropriate treatment approach and some research has been undertaken in the area. For the present there is no immediate resolution of the balance of risks and benefits. It seems sensible to have a cautious approach to using combination DMARDs in these patients.

References

1. Gaujoux-Viala C, Nam J, Ramiro S, Landewe R, Buch MH, Smolen JS, et al. Efficacy of conventional synthetic disease-modifying antirheumatic drugs, glucocorticoids and tofacitinib: a systematic literature review informing the 2013 update of the EULAR recommendations for management of rheumatoid arthritis. Ann Rheum Dis. 2014;73:510–5.
2. van Gestel AM, Haagsma CJ, Furst DE, van Riel PL. Treatment of early rheumatoid arthritis patients with slow-acting anti-rheumatic drugs (SAARDs). Baillieres Clin Rheumatol. 1997;11:65–82.
3. Donahue KE, Gartlehner G, Jonas DE, Lux LJ, Thieda P, Jonas BL, et al. Systematic review: comparative effectiveness and harms of disease-modifying medications for rheumatoid arthritis. Ann Intern Med. 2008;148:124–34.
4. Chakravarty K, McDonald H, Pullar T, Taggart A, Chalmers R, Oliver S, et al. BSR/BHPR guideline for disease-modifying anti-rheumatic drug (DMARD) therapy in consultation with the British Association of Dermatologists. Rheumatology (Oxford). 2008;47:924–5.
5. O'Mahony R, Richards A, Deighton C, Scott D. Withdrawal of disease-modifying antirheumatic drugs in patients with rheumatoid arthritis: a systematic review and meta-analysis. Ann Rheum Dis. 2010;69:1823–6.
6. Agarwal S, Zaman T, Handa R. Retention rates of disease-modifying anti-rheumatic drugs in patients with rheumatoid arthritis. Singapore Med J. 2009;50:686–92.
7. Solomon DH, Bitton A, Katz JN, Radner H, Brown EM, Fraenkel L. Review: treat to target in rheumatoid arthritis: fact, fiction, or hypothesis? Arthritis Rheum. 2014;66:775–82.
8. Huynh D, Kavanaugh A. Psoriatic arthritis: current therapy and future approaches. Rheumatology (Oxford). 2015;54:20–8.
9. Yang Z, Zhao W, Liu W, Lv Q, Dong X. Efficacy evaluation of methotrexate in the treatment of ankylosing spondylitis using meta-analysis. Int J Clin Pharmacol Ther. 2014;52:346–51.

10. Smolen JS, Kalden JR, Scott DL, Rozman B, Kvien TK, Larsen A, et al. Efficacy and safety of leflunomide compared with placebo and sulphasalazine in active rheumatoid arthritis: a double-blind, randomised, multicentre trial. European Leflunomide Study Group. Lancet. 1999;353:259–66.

11. Cohen S, Cannon GW, Schiff M, Weaver A, Fox R, Olsen N, et al. Two-year, blinded, randomized, controlled trial of treatment of active rheumatoid arthritis with leflunomide compared with methotrexate. Utilization of Leflunomide in the Treatment of Rheumatoid Arthritis Trial Investigator Group. Arthritis Rheum. 2001;44:1984–92.

12. Strand V, Cohen S, Schiff M, Weaver A, Fleischmann R, Cannon G, et al. Treatment of active rheumatoid arthritis with leflunomide compared with placebo and methotrexate. Leflunomide Rheumatoid Arthritis Investigators Group. Arch Intern Med. 1999;159:2542–50.

13. Scott DL, Strand V. The effects of disease-modifying anti-rheumatic drugs on the Health Assessment Questionnaire score. Lessons from the leflunomide clinical trials database. Rheumatology (Oxford). 2002;41:899–909.

14. Jones G, Halbert J, Crotty M, Shanahan EM, Batterham M, Ahern M. The effect of treatment on radiological progression in rheumatoid arthritis: a systematic review of randomized placebo-controlled trials. Rheumatology (Oxford). 2003;42:6–13.

15. Favalli EG, Biggioggero M, Meroni PL. Methotrexate for the treatment of rheumatoid arthritis in the biologic era: still an "anchor" drug? Autoimmun Rev. 2014;13:1102–8.

16. Braun J, Kastner P, Flaxenberg P, Wahrisch J, Hanke P, Demary W, et al. Comparison of the clinical efficacy and safety of subcutaneous versus oral administration of methotrexate in patients with active rheumatoid arthritis: results of a six-month, multi-center, randomized, double-blind, controlled, phase IV trial. Arthritis Rheum. 2008;58:73–81.

17. Pincus T, Castrejon I. Evidence that the strategy is more important than the agent to treat rheumatoid arthritis. Data from clinical trials of combinations of non-biologic DMARDs, with protocol-driven intensification of therapy for tight control or treat-to-target. Bull Hosp Jt Dis. 2013;71 Suppl 1:S33–40.

18. Bijlsma JW. Disease control with glucocorticoid therapy in rheumatoid arthritis. Rheumatology (Oxford). 2012;51 Suppl 4:iv9–13.

19. Ma MH, Kingsley GH, Scott DL. A systematic comparison of combination DMARD therapy and tumour necrosis inhibitor therapy with methotrexate in patients with early rheumatoid arthritis. Rheumatology (Oxford). 2010;49:91–8.

Chapter 7
Biologics – An Overview

Abstract   The biologics used in inflammatory arthritis are genetically engineered proteins derived from human genes. They inhibit specific components of the immune system, which play pivotal roles in driving or inhibiting inflammation in arthritis. Unlike conventional drugs that modify the immune system as a whole, biologics affect specific components of the immune system. Theoretically this targeted approach is both more specific in its effects and causes fewer adverse events. However, in reality the complex interactions of cytokines and the multiplicity of cytokine targets means it is difficult to predict the effectiveness and toxicity of cytokine-based interventions such as biologics. There are currently six different classes of biologics available for the treatment of inflammatory arthritis patients. Each inhibits a different aspect of the immune driven inflammatory pathway. This chapter will provide a broad overview of the available biologics, the current treatment pathways dictating their prescribing in the UK and the health economics issues surrounding their use.

Keywords   Biologics • Anti-TNF • Rituximab • Tocilizumab • Abatacept • Side-Effects

I.C. Scott et al., *Inflammatory Arthritis in Clinical Practice*,
DOI 10.1007/978-1-4471-6648-1_7,
© Springer-Verlag London 2015

Introduction

A biologic therapy, simply put, is a treatment that has been derived from a biological process rather than being manufactured chemically. In medical terms, this includes blood products, vaccinations and, more recently, monoclonal antibodies (often called "biologics").

Historically, long term outcomes in RA were considered not to be modifiable [1]. The introduction of biologic drugs has resulted in a complete shift of the goal posts of therapy. Conventional anti- rheumatic drugs such as DMARDs are small molecules that are designed to bind to and interfere with a target receptor. However, a key challenge with a small molecule agent is a lack of specificity. Methotrexate, for example, targets multiple immune pathways including neutrophils, B cells and T cells. The idea of a 'magic bullet' approach to target one specific immune process has long been the goal of drug development in RA.

In the late 1990s Elliot et al. published a phase 2 trial of the compound cA2, a monoclonal antibody later to be named infliximab, targeting tumour necrosis factor (TNF) in patients with RA [2]. Elliot's study revealed results that were unparalleled in the field, with 2/24 patients in the placebo responding, compared to 19/24 in those treated with 10 mg/kg of the study drug. Infliximab moved into phase three trials producing equally optimistic results [3]. Since the success of the first anti-TNF, multiple other monoclonal antibodies have been licensed for the treatment of RA. There are now numerous anti-TNF agents, as well as monoclonal antibodies targeting interleukins, B cells and T cells.

The biologics used in inflammatory arthritis are genetically engineered proteins derived from human genes. They inhibit specific components of the immune system which play pivotal roles in driving or inhibiting inflammation in arthritis. Unlike conventional drugs, that modify the immune system as a whole, biologics affect specific components of the immune system. Theoretically this targeted approach is both more specific in its effects and causes fewer adverse events.

However, in reality the complex interactions of cytokines and the multiplicity of cytokine targets means it is difficult to predict the effectiveness and toxicity of cytokine-based interventions such as biologics. Several strategies have been explored to treat inflammatory diseases with cytokines. These include neutralizing cytokines using soluble receptors or monoclonal antibodies, receptor blockade, and the activation of anti-inflammatory pathways by bioengineered versions of immunoregulatory cytokines.

There are currently six different classes of biologics available for the treatment of inflammatory arthritis (Table 7.1).

TABLE 7.1 Currently available biologic agents for the treatment of inflammatory arthritis

Biologic type	Therapeutic agent(s)	Target disease(s)
TNF-inhibitors	Adalimumab	RA/AS/PsA
	Etanercept	RA/AS/PsA
	Infliximab	RA/PsA[a]
	Certolizumab	RA/AS[a]/PsA[a]
	Golimumab	RA/AS/PsA
Interleukin-1 receptor inhibition	Anakinra	RA[a]
B-cell inhibition	Rituximab	RA
T-cell inhibition	Abatacept	RA
Interleukin-6 inhibition	Tocilizumab	RA
Interleukin-12/-23 inhibition	Ustekinumab	PsA[a]

RA Rheumatoid Arthritis, AS Ankylosing Spondylitis, PsA Psoriatic Arthritis

[a]Not currently approved by the National Institute for Health and Care Excellence (NICE)

Each inhibits a different aspect of the immune driven inflammatory pathway. These biologic classes comprise:

- TNF-inhibitors, of which five biologics are currently available
- Interleukin-1 receptor inhibition, with one biologic currently available
- B-cell inhibition, with one biologic currently available
- T-cell inhibition, with one biologic currently available
- Interleukin-6 inhibition, with one biologic currently available
- Interleukin-12/-23 inhibition, with one biologic currently available

Most of the new biologics that followed TNF-inhibitors are focused on patients who have failed these agents. It is considered inappropriate to combine biologics and the balance of evidence suggests there may be increased toxicity without enhanced benefit from combination of biologics.

Biologic Treatment Pathways

Rheumatoid Arthritis

With the exception of Ustekinumab, all the available biologics have been shown in clinical trials to effectively treat RA. The initial agent of choice is usually a TNF-inhibitor. The use of biologics in the UK is restricted by the National Institute for Health and Care Excellence (NICE) to patients who have failed two conventional DMARDs, including methotrexate and have active disease defined as having a DAS28 score >5.1 on two occasions 1 month apart [4]. The figure below outlines the current biologic treatment paradigm for RA in the UK (Fig. 7.1). There is growing evidence to favour certain agents in specific clinical circumstances. These issues will be discussed in more detail in subsequent chapters.

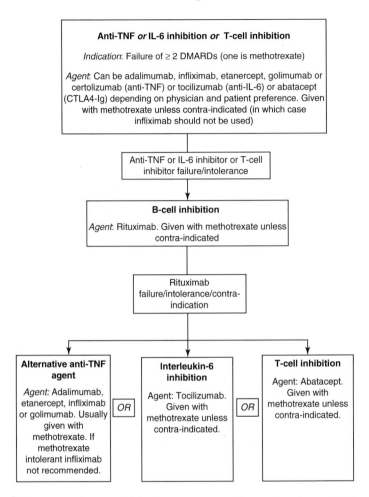

FIGURE 7.1 Current biologic treatment pathway for rheumatoid arthritis in the UK (Figure reproduced with permission from Scott [5] licensed under the Creative Commons Attribution License)

Early Rheumatoid Arthritis

Biologics are especially effective in early RA, particularly when combined with methotrexate [6]. Currently, their cost has restricted their use in this situation. Whether or not this is correct is an issue for governments and health care funders rather than for clinicians and patients. The evidence for efficacy in early disease is strong but the evidence for their being cost-effective in this situation is controversial.

Psoriatic Arthritis

TNF inhibitors are effective in PsA. Their use is restricted under NICE to patients with peripheral arthritis involving three or more joints which are swollen and tender who have failed at least two standard DMARDs. They improve both the arthritis and the skin disease. Patients with psoriatic spondyloarthritis in whom spinal disease is the dominant problem should be treated as per patients with AS (see below). The newer biologic agent, Ustekinumab has been shown to be effective for PsA. Although it is approved by NICE for the treatment of skin psoriasis it has not yet been recommended for the treatment of PsA.

Ankylosing Spondylitis

TNF inhibitors are effective in AS and improve the spinal disease as well as any peripheral arthritis. They are indicated in patients with a score of at least four units on the Bath Ankylosing Spondylitis Disease Activity Index (BASDAI) and at least 4 cm on a 10 cm spinal pain visual analogue scale. Patients should also have failed to respond to conventional treatment with two or more non-steroidal anti-inflammatory drugs taken sequentially. Patients should show a response to anti-TNF therapy with a reduction of the BASDAI score to 50 % of the pre-treatment value or by two or more units and reduced spinal pain on the VAS by 2 cm or more. There is evidence that etanercept and adalimumab are more cost effective than infliximab in AS, with the latter agent not being recommended for routine use in the UK.

Health Economic Case for Using Biologics

The biologics are both safe and effective treatments but they are also very expensive. If cost did not enter the equation, these agents would be the most likely first choice treatment for most patients. However, whilst treatment with conventional DMARD costs such as methotrexate is inexpensive, the costs of biologics are far higher. No matter how good these new treatments prove to be, their use is bound to be restricted by costs.

On the other side of the equation is the high cost and disadvantages of RA for both the patient and for society as a whole. The argument about when to use these new drugs and their relative cost-effectiveness is complex. At present it is thought that it is reasonably cost-effective to use them in patients with active disease who have failed to respond to a number of conventional DMARDs.

Decisions about the use of high cost treatments are based on cost-utility analyses, which is a key pharmacoeconomic issue. It estimates the ratio between the cost of a health-related intervention, such as a new biologic, and its benefit in terms of the number of years lived in full health by the beneficiaries. It is a special case of a cost-effectiveness analysis. Costs is measured in monetary units. However, benefits are described in a way that lets health states considered less preferable to full health to be given quantitative values. This is usually as quality-adjusted life years (QALYs). The incremental cost-effectiveness ratio is the ratio between the difference in costs and the difference in benefits of two interventions. A threshold value is often set by policy makers. In the UK the threshold is about £20–30,000 per QALY. Health interventions that have an incremental cost of more than £30,000 per additional QALY gained are likely to be rejected and an intervention which has an incremental cost of less than or equal to £30,000 per extra QALY gained is likely to be accepted as cost-effective. In North America US$50,000 per QALY is often suggested as a threshold for a cost-effective intervention.

This seems simple and non-controversial. However, the mechanisms for assessing the QALYs gained by using high cost treatments like biologics in long-term diseases such as RA are highly controversial. The same data is used by different experts to produce highly different results. One particular reason for these difficulties is that although the costs of a drug are uniform the costs of treatment are not spread equally between patients; most patients incur relatively low costs but a small number of patients have very high costs. The same is true of health benefits. As a consequence the issues about access to biologics remain debatable.

References

1. Scott DL, Symmons DP, Coulton BL, Popert AJ. Long-term outcome of treating rheumatoid arthritis: results after 20 years. Lancet. 1987;1:1108–11.
2. Elliott MJ, Maini RN, Feldmann M, Kalden JR, Antoni C, Smolen JS, et al. Randomised double-blind comparison of chimeric monoclonal antibody to tumour necrosis factor alpha (cA2) versus placebo in rheumatoid arthritis. Lancet. 1994;344:1105–10.
3. Lipsky PE, van der Heijde DM, St Clair EW, Furst DE, Breedveld FC, Kalden JR, et al. Infliximab and methotrexate in the treatment of rheumatoid arthritis. Anti-Tumor Necrosis Factor Trial in Rheumatoid Arthritis with Concomitant Therapy Study Group. N Engl J Med. 2000;343:1594–602.
4. National Institute for Health and Care Excellence. Adalimumab, etanercept and infliximab for the treatment of rheumatoid arthritis. NICE Website. 2007. http://www.nice.org.uk/TA130. Accessed 20 Apr 2014.
5. Scott IC. Risk prediction in rheumatoid arthritis. Unpublished thesis, King's College London; 2014.
6. Breedveld FC, Weisman MH, Kavanaugh AF, Cohen SB, Pavelka K, van Vollenhoven R, et al. The PREMIER study: a multicenter, randomized, double-blind clinical trial of combination therapy with adalimumab plus methotrexate versus methotrexate alone or adalimumab alone in patients with early, aggressive rheumatoid arthritis who had not had previous methotrexate treatment. Arthritis Rheum. 2006;54:26–37.

Chapter 8
Anti-Tumour Necrosis Factor-Alpha (TNF-α) Treatment

Abstract There are currently five TNF-α inhibitors available to treat inflammatory arthropathies. These can be subdivided into first generation agents (comprising etanercept, infliximab and adalimumab) and second generation agents (comprising certolizumab and golimumab). In RA all TNF-α inhibitors are nationally approved for use in routine clinical care. There is no evidence that one of these agents is superior to another and practical and financial issues determine which is chosen. In other forms of inflammatory arthritis, in particular in AS, there is evidence that some biologics may be less effective than others. Overall, there is strong clinical trial evidence for their efficacy in inflammatory arthritis. Although relatively safe, TNF-α inhibitors have a broad range of potential adverse effects. The dominant risk is an increased infection risk, particularly that of latent tuberculosis reactivation. This chapter will provide an overview of the available TNF-α inhibitors, their mechanisms of action, the evidence base for their efficacy and the potential adverse events associated with them.

Keywords TNF-α • Etanercept • Infliximab • Adalimumab • Certolizumab • Golimumab • Side-Effects • Tuberculosis

I.C. Scott et al., *Inflammatory Arthritis in Clinical Practice*,
DOI 10.1007/978-1-4471-6648-1_8,
© Springer-Verlag London 2015

Background

Early research in the 1980s and 1990s highlighted the importance of cytokines in inflammatory arthritis. It showed many different pro- and anti-inflammatory cytokines were over-expressed in the rheumatoid synovium. Although there was debate about whether IL-1 was the major driver in inflammatory arthritis, research suggested that TNF-α might have a central role. The proof of principle for inhibiting this cytokine came from an open label clinical study in which patients with RA received a single infusion of a TNF-α inhibitor. This showed a rapid response, including an early fall in CRP levels [1]. However, the anti-inflammatory effect lasted only 6–12 weeks. It was followed by a return of active disease. As a result patients were retreated with further infusions and they showed responses of a similar magnitude and duration. The scene was set for a major clinical development programme. One concern was that the TNF-α inhibitor, which included mouse protein, might lose efficacy due to immunogenicity. Up to 60 % of Infliximab treated patients develop anti-drug antibodies [2]. This was solved by giving methotrexate as an additional treatment. This has become a standard approach with these biologics.

There are currently five TNF-α inhibitors available to treat inflammatory arthropathies (Table 8.1). These can be subdivided into first generation agents (comprising etanercept, infliximab and adalimumab) and second generation agents (comprising certolizumab and golimumab). In RA all TNF-α inhibitors are nationally approved for use in routine clinical care. There is no evidence that one of these agents is superior to another, and practical and financial issues determine which is chosen. In other forms of inflammatory arthritis, in particular in AS, there is evidence that some biologics may be less effective than others.

Table 8.1 Currently available TNF-α inhibitors for the treatment of inflammatory arthritis

TNF-α inhibitor	Site of action	Dosing schedule	Methotrexate
Infliximab	Binds soluble and transmembrane TNF-α and inhibits binding of TNF-α to TNF receptors	IV administration every 4–8 weeks	Essential to co-prescribe
Etanercept	Soluble TNF-receptor fusion protein that binds TNF-α and TNF-β preventing them from interacting with their receptors	Subcutaneous once or twice weekly	Optional to co-prescribe
Adalimumab	Binds soluble and transmembrane TNF-α and inhibits binding of TNF-α to TNF receptors	Subcutaneous fortnightly	Optional to co-prescribe
Certolizumab	Binds soluble and transmembrane TNF-α and inhibits binding of TNF-α to TNF receptors	Subcutaneous fortnightly	Optional to co-prescribe
Golimumab	Binds soluble and transmembrane TNF-α and inhibits binding of TNF-α to TNF receptors	Subcutaneously monthly	Optional to co-prescribe

Etanercept

Etanercept is a soluble TNF-receptor fusion protein. It comprises two dimers. Each dimer has an extracellular, ligand-binding portion of the higher-affinity type 2 TNF receptor (p75) which is linked to the Fc portion of human IgG1. This fusion protein binds to both TNF-α and TNF-β and prevents them from interacting with their receptors. It is given by subcutaneous administration at a dose of 25 mg twice a week or 50 mg once a week. This dosing reflects its half-life of approximately 4 days. Interestingly etanercept has never received a license for inflammatory bowel disease because of lack of efficacy in clinical trials [3].

Infliximab

Infliximab is a chimeric IgG1 anti–TNF-α antibody in which the antigen-binding region is derived from a mouse antibody and the constant region from a human antibody. It binds to soluble and membrane bound TNF-α with high affinity. This binding impairs the binding of TNF-α to its receptor. Infliximab also kills cells that express TNF-α through antibody- dependent and complement-dependent cytotoxicity. There are considerable differences between patients in the pharmacokinetics of infliximab. The intravenous dosing method of infliximab results in much greater initial peak concentrations along with higher peak to trough ratios when compared to other anti-TNF agents [4]. Trough concentrations, seen 8 weeks after intravenous administration of 3 mg/kg of infliximab vary enormously between patients. Shortening the interval between doses may be more effective in increasing the trough levels than increasing the dose. In RA patients the dose given is 3 mg/kg every 8 weeks. In PsA and AS the dose is 5 mg/kg every 8 weeks. Some patients have higher doses, and in certain circumstances the intervals between doses can be reduced.

Adalimumab

This is a recombinant human IgG1 monoclonal antibody. It binds human TNF-α with a high affinity, and as a consequence inhibits this cytokine binding to its receptors. It also lyses cells that express TNF-*a* on their surface. It is given by subcutaneous injection and is then absorbed slowly. Peak concentrations are achieved after 120 h. Although there are wide variations between patients, it is given fortnightly at a dose of 40 mg.

Certolizumab

Certolizumab pegol is a recombinant humanised Fab fragment (which is the antigen-binding domain) of a TNF-α antibody, which has been coupled to polyethylene glycol (PEG). This coupling prolongs its plasma half-life to approximately 2 weeks. It binds and neutralises membrane-bound and soluble human TNF-α. It is the only TNF-α inhibitor without an Fc region. It is given by subcutaneous injection with an initial "loading dose" of 400 mg every 2 weeks for 6 weeks, followed by 200 mg once fortnightly.

Golimumab

Golimumab is a human IgG1 monoclonal antibody against TNF-α, which is produced in a transgenic mouse. It targets and neutralises both soluble and membrane bound TNF-α. It has a variable half-life of between 7 and 20 days. It is given as a monthly subcutaneous injection at dose of 50 mg, which can be increased to 100 mg a month if the patient's body-weight is more than 100 kg.

Indications

Rheumatoid Arthritis

TNF-α inhibitors should be initiated when patients continue to have active RA (defined as a DAS28 score of >5.1 on two occasions at least 1 month apart) after an adequate trial of effective DMARDs (defined as 6 months of treatment with at least 2 DMARDs, one of which must be methotrexate). Unless contra-indicated they are given with methotrexate, which increases efficacy and helps to prevent the formation of anti-biologic antibodies. Their use as the first line for the treatment of RA should at present be limited to research studies.

Psoriatic Arthritis

As with RA, TNF-α inhibitors in PsA are restricted to patients who continue to have active disease despite DMARD therapy. Current national guidelines recommend their use in patients with active PsA (defined as a tender and swollen joint count of at least 3) despite treatment with two DMARDs (given for 6 months, one of which is methotrexate).

Ankylosing Spondylitis

TNF-α inhibitors are of proven efficacy in AS. They are used in patients who have not responded to treatment with NSAIDs. NSAID failure is defined as an inability of NSAID drugs taken sequentially at maximum tolerated doses for 4 weeks to control symptoms. Patients require active disease with a BASDAI score of at least four units and a spinal pain VAS of at least 4 cm.

Clinical Effects

Rheumatoid Arthritis

TNF-α inhibitors given in adequate doses produce major improvements in symptoms, signs, and laboratory measures. This improvement occurs within 12 weeks of starting treatment. Switching from one TNF-α inhibitor to another is well documented, with supporting evidence from clinical trials.

Individually important responses should occur within 8–12 weeks. Provided there is some evidence of benefit, treatment should be continued. If patients show no response therapy should be altered. In patients with an incomplete response, there is some evidence that increasing the dose or reducing dosing intervals may provide additional benefit, as may the addition or substitution of other DMARDs.

A systematic review of the efficacy of TNF-α inhibitors in RA showed the number needed to treat was 5 to obtain an ACR20 response and 7 to obtain an ACR70 response

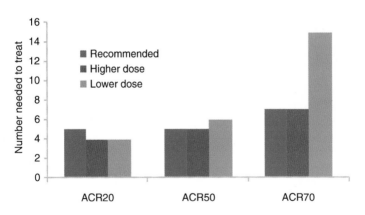

FIGURE 8.1   Number needed to treat for ACR20 to ACR70 responses with TNF-α inhibitors in rheumatoid arthritis (Figure adapted using data reported by Alonso-Ruiz et al. [5])

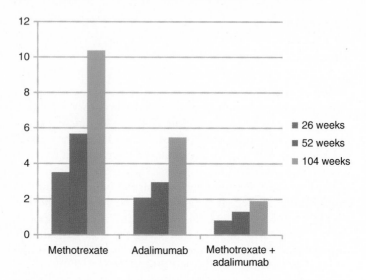

Figure 8.2 Mean changes from baseline in X-Ray (sharp) scores over 104 weeks in the PREMIER study evaluating methotrexate monotherapy, adalimumab monotherapy or double therapy with both medications (Figure adapted using data reported by Breedveld et al. [6])

(Fig. 8.1) [5]. Clinical features like joint counts, disability and joint damage were all improved or progressed less with TNF-α inhibitor use. There was no reason to prefer one TNF-α inhibitor over another. There was limited evidence that giving lower or higher doses changes the effect of biologics, though lower doses reduced the chance of developing an ACR70 response.

There is growing evidence that TNF-α inhibitors slow radiographic progression in RA (Fig. 8.2) [6]. In some patients they completely halt it. The evidence is stronger in early disease. It is also stronger with combined therapy using methotrexate with a biologic. The relationship between clinical and radiological response is incomplete. However, the long term implications of slowing radiological damage are uncertain, and benefits on radiological damage alone should not influence clinical decision making.

Psoriatic Arthritis

Infliximab, etanercept and adalimumab have all been effective in clinical trials. A meta-analysis in 2008 evaluated 6 RCTs in which these TNF-α inhibitors had been used [7]. Nine hundred and eighty two patients were enrolled. All three anti-TNF agents were significantly more effective at treating PsA compared with placebo. Patients treated with biologics were 4 times more likely to attain an ACR20 response, 10 times more likely to attain ACR50 response and 17 times more likely to attain an ACR70 response when compared with placebo.

The GO-REVEAL study showed the efficacy of golimumab in treating PsA [8]. After 14 weeks of treatment in this RCT 51 % of patients receiving 50 mg of golimumab once monthly and 45 % of patients receiving 100 mg of golimumab once monthly attained an ACR 20 response compared with 9 % of patients in the placebo group ($p < 0.001$).

These agents have the additional important benefit of being able to effectively treat the skin disease concurrently with joint symptoms and signs.

Ankylosing Spondylitis

The TNF-α inhibitors infliximab, etanercept and adalimumab have proven efficacy for the treatment of AS. A systematic review and meta-analysis of 8 RCTs found that treatment with TNF-α inhibitors provided standardized mean differences (95 % CI) of −0.9 (−1.07, −0.73) for pain measured by spinal pain VAS, and −1.25 (−1.51, −0.98) for disease activity measured by the BASDAI [9].

Safety and Adverse Effects

Biologics Registries

Much data exists on the safety of TNF-α inhibitors. Several international biologic registries have been compiled, which have examined the adverse effects of these agents in large numbers of RA patients receiving biologics compared with matched controls not receiving biologics. These comprise the British Society for Rheumatology Biologics Register (BSRBR; United Kingdom), the Rheumatoid Arthritis-Observation of Biologic Therapy Register (RABBIT; Germany) and the Spanish Registry of Adverse Events of Biological Therapies in Rheumatic Diseases (BIOBADASER; Spain). The majority of data are on first-generation agents with limited information on second-line agents. There is however little evidence to suggest they have significantly different complication rates.

Local Injection Site Reactions

Local reactions such as minor redness and itching at the injection site are common with subcutaneously administered biologics. They last a few days.

Hypersensitivity Responses

Minor symptoms such as headache and nausea are common in patients during infliximab infusions. Symptoms suggesting an immediate hypersensitivity response with infliximab infusions, such as urticaria, are uncommon but well described; serious anaphylaxis is rare. Antihistamines, steroids and adrenaline should be available while infusions are being given, though they are rarely needed.

Infections

Serious and opportunistic infections occur in patients receiving TNF-α inhibitors. Examples of such infections include septic arthritis, infected prostheses, acute abscesses and osteomyelitis. Until recently it was unclear if the incidence of these infections on TNF-α inhibitors exceeded that of patients with severe RA, who are twice as likely to develop serious infection compared with the general population. The biologic registries have however indicated that TNF-α inhibitor use is associated with an approximate doubling in the risk of serious infection. This risk is especially prominent in the first 6 months of treatment. Analysis of data from the BSRBR found that the adjusted hazard ratio (HR) for serious infections on TNF-α inhibitors compared with standard DMARDs was 1.2 (95 % confidence interval 1.1, 1.5); in the first 6 months of treatment this was higher at 1.8 (95 % confidence interval 1.3, 2.6) [10]. If serious infections develop then these agents should be withheld until it has resolved as there is some evidence that they worsen infection if continued.

Tuberculosis is a particular concern. TNF-α is integral in maintaining the integrity of formed TB granulomas. There is both an increased susceptibility to primary tuberculosis and, more importantly, reactivation of latent tuberculosis. Screening patients for tuberculosis reduces the risk of activating tuberculosis and it is recommended that all patients should be evaluated for the possibility of latent tuberculosis. This evaluation should include a detailed history and examination, together with screening tests, such as skin tests/ interferon-gamma release assays and chest radiography, depending on current national recommendations. Treatment for the possibility of latent tuberculosis should be considered if patients may be at risk. Some experts consider TNF-α inhibitors may be started as soon as anti-tuberculosis chemotherapy is started, although there is debate on the best timing. Not all TNF-α inhibitors carry the same risk of TB with the risk being substantially higher with infliximab and adalimumab than etanercept [11]. Additionally the onset of TB development varies between agents with TB infection manifesting in the early stages of treatment with infliximab but occurring relatively evenly throughout the period of etanercept treatment. The risk with the second generation TNF-α inhibitors is currently unclear due to limited experience with these newer agents.

Demyelinating-like Disorders

Demyelinating-like disorders of both the peripheral and central nervous systems alongside optic neuritis have been reported in patients receiving TNF-α inhibitors. Cases of peripheral nerve demyelination such as Guillain-Barré syndrome and chronic inflammatory demyelinating polyneuropathy have been reported. In most instances withdrawal of the offending drug resulted in slow symptom improvement however a minority of individuals never achieved full symptom resolution. Both exacerbations of previously quiescent multiple sclerosis and new-onset demyelinating diseases have been reported. These agents should be stopped if a demyelinating-like disorder or optic neuritis occurs and patients with a history of definite multiple sclerosis should not receive TNF-α inhibitors.

Haematological Disorders

A few cases of pancytopenia and aplastic anaemia have been reported. If these problems occur, treatment should be stopped and patients evaluated for underlying diseases or other causative drugs. No monitoring is currently recommended as these are rare events.

Heart Failure

Although heart failure is associated with high levels of TNF-α, several clinical trials examining infliximab and etanercept as treatments for heart failure found a trend towards worsening cardiac congestion in patients receiving these biologics [12, 13]. They were however used in higher doses than are routinely prescribed in RA patients. For this reason current guidelines recommend anti-TNF therapy should be used with caution in patients with mild heart failure (defined as class I or II New York Heart Association heart failure) and avoided in those with significant heart failure (defined as class III or IV New York Heart Association heart failure). If cardiac failure develops or worsens with treatment then anti-TNF therapy should be withdrawn.

Malignancy

There is no definitive evidence that anti-TNF treatments increase the risk of either lymphoproliferative disorders or solid malignancies. Although lymphoma has been reported it remains uncertain whether this is a causal relationship because the incidence of lymphoma is increased in patients with RA irrespective of treatments. Additionally the types of lymphoma in RA patients and those reported in patients given TNF-α inhibitors are similar. There is however evidence for an increased risk of skin cancers in patients treated with anti-TNF [14]. There is a paucity of available data on cancer recurrence in patients in remission from previous malignancies receiving TNF-α inhibitors however caution in using these agents is advisable due to the role of TNF-α in immune surveillance for cancer.

Auto-immune Disorders

The auto-antibodies, anti-nuclear antibody (ANA) and double stranded DNA antibody (dsDNA) are reported to occur relatively often in patients receiving anti-TNF therapy. ANA is estimated to occur in up to 52 % of RA patients. These are commoner with infliximab. The occurrence of clinically overt drug-induced lupus or vasculitis is however rare. In patients who develop anti-TNF related lupus the clinical features differ from classical drug-induced lupus with higher rates of cerebral and renal involvement that is similar to mild idiopathic SLE. Withdrawal of the agent usually results in symptom resolution although steroids or alternative immunosuppressives are occasionally required.

Interstitial Lung Disease

Interstitial lung disease (ILD) has been reported to occur with all first generation TNF-α inhibitors. It is however difficult to establish a causative relationship in RA patients because ILD is a well recognised extra-articular manifestation of RA. Current recommendations are that patients with known ILD should receive close lung function monitoring and if worsening or new ILD features develop consideration should be given to stopping therapy [15].

Psoriasis

Although anti-TNF is used to treat psoriasis there has emerged a significant number of cases of de-novo psoriasis developing in patients receiving all first-generation agents. Stopping the TNF-α inhibitor often improves the skin disease, although skin specific therapies may be needed.

Immune Responses to TNF-α Inhibitors

Patients may develop antibiologic antibodies. This is relevant in those receiving infliximab where such antibodies may accelerate its clearance, increase the risk of infusion reactions and reduce responses. Higher doses of infliximab and concomitant methotrexate administration reduce the occurrence of human anti-chimeric antibody responses [16]. The experience with adalimumab reveals lower rates of immunogenicity, but with immunogenicity responses correlating to reduced efficacy [17]. Antibodies to other anti-TNF agents can also occur however their clinical significance is uncertain.

Switching Anti-TNF Agents in Cases of Primary or Secondary Failure

A substantial proportion of patients fail to respond to anti-TNF therapy. Up to one third of patients discontinue anti-TNF therapy within 1 year due to insufficient responses (termed primary failure) or a loss of efficacy (termed secondary failure). In such cases current guidance suggests that rituximab should be initiated as a second line therapy. However in cases of rituximab failure or contra-indication it is reasonable to try an alternative anti-TNF agent. Studies have shown that clinical improvements following the switch to a second TNF-α inhibitor are similar to those seen in RA patients receiving their first anti-TNF agent. Clinical responses are however diminished in individuals needing a third anti-TNF drug. Responses are also superior in cases of secondary compared with primary failure, which suggests the cytokine pathways driving RA differ between individuals [18].

References

1. Elliott MJ, Maini RN, Feldmann M, Kalden JR, Antoni C, Smolen JS, et al. Randomised double-blind comparison of chimeric monoclonal antibody to tumour necrosis factor alpha (cA2) versus placebo in rheumatoid arthritis. Lancet. 1994;344: 1105–10.
2. Maini R, St Clair EW, Breedveld F, Furst D, Kalden J, Weisman M, et al. Infliximab (chimeric anti-tumour necrosis factor alpha monoclonal antibody) versus placebo in rheumatoid arthritis patients receiving concomitant methotrexate: a randomised phase III trial. ATTRACT Study Group. Lancet. 1999;354: 1932–9.
3. Sandborn WJ, Hanauer SB, Katz S, Safdi M, Wolf DG, Baerg RD, et al. Etanercept for active Crohn's disease: a randomized, double-blind, placebo-controlled trial. Gastroenterology. 2001;121:1088–94.
4. Nestorov I. Clinical pharmacokinetics of tumor necrosis factor antagonists. J Rheumatol Suppl. 2005;74:13–8.
5. Alonso-Ruiz A, Pijoan JI, Ansuategui E, Urkaregi A, Calabozo M, Quintana A. Tumor necrosis factor alpha drugs in rheumatoid arthritis: systematic review and metaanalysis of efficacy and safety. BMC Musculoskelet Disord. 2008;9:52.
6. Breedveld FC, Weisman MH, Kavanaugh AF, Cohen SB, Pavelka K, van Vollenhoven R, et al. The PREMIER study: a multicenter, randomized, double-blind clinical trial of combination therapy with adalimumab plus methotrexate versus methotrexate alone or adalimumab alone in patients with early, aggressive rheumatoid arthritis who had not had previous methotrexate treatment. Arthritis Rheum. 2006;54:26–37.

7. Saad AA, Symmons DP, Noyce PR, Ashcroft DM. Risks and benefits of tumor necrosis factor-alpha inhibitors in the management of psoriatic arthritis: systematic review and metaanalysis of randomized controlled trials. J Rheumatol. 2008;35:883–90.

8. Kavanaugh A, van der Heijde D, McInnes IB, Mease P, Krueger GG, Gladman DD, et al. Golimumab in psoriatic arthritis: one-year clinical efficacy, radiographic, and safety results from a phase III, randomized, placebo-controlled trial. Arthritis Rheum. 2012;64:2504–17.

9. Escalas C, Trijau S, Dougados M. Evaluation of the treatment effect of NSAIDs/TNF blockers according to different domains in ankylosing spondylitis: results of a meta-analysis. Rheumatology (Oxford). 2010;49:1317–25.

10. Galloway JB, Hyrich KL, Mercer LK, Dixon WG, Fu B, Ustianowski AP, et al. Anti-TNF therapy is associated with an increased risk of serious infections in patients with rheumatoid arthritis especially in the first 6 months of treatment: updated results from the British Society for Rheumatology Biologics Register with special emphasis on risks in the elderly. Rheumatology (Oxford). 2011;50:124–31.

11. Dixon WG, Hyrich KL, Watson KD, Lunt M, Galloway J, Ustianowski A, et al. Drug-specific risk of tuberculosis in patients with rheumatoid arthritis treated with anti-TNF therapy: results from the British Society for Rheumatology Biologics Register (BSRBR). Ann Rheum Dis. 2010;69:522–8.

12. Bozkurt B, Torre-Amione G, Warren MS, Whitmore J, Soran OZ, Feldman AM, et al. Results of targeted anti-tumor necrosis factor therapy with etanercept (ENBREL) in patients with advanced heart failure. Circulation. 2001;103:1044–7.

13. Chung ES, Packer M, Lo KH, Fasanmade AA, Willerson JT, Anti TNFTACHFI. Randomized, double-blind, placebo-controlled, pilot trial of infliximab, a chimeric monoclonal antibody to tumor necrosis factor-alpha, in patients with moderate-to-severe heart failure: results of the anti-TNF Therapy Against Congestive Heart Failure (ATTACH) trial. Circulation. 2003;107:3133–40.

14. Mariette X, Reynolds AV, Emery P. Updated meta-analysis of non-melanoma skin cancer rates reported from prospective observational studies in patients treated with tumour necrosis factor inhibitors. Ann Rheum Dis. 2012;71:e2.

15. Jani M, Hirani N, Matteson EL, Dixon WG. The safety of biologic therapies in RA-associated interstitial lung disease. Nat Rev Rheumatol. 2014;10:284–94.
16. Maini RN, Breedveld FC, Kalden JR, Smolen JS, Davis D, Macfarlane JD, et al. Therapeutic efficacy of multiple intravenous infusions of anti-tumor necrosis factor alpha monoclonal antibody combined with low-dose weekly methotrexate in rheumatoid arthritis. Arthritis Rheum. 1998;41:1552–63.
17. Bartelds GM, Wijbrandts CA, Nurmohamed MT, Stapel S, Lems WF, Aarden L, et al. Clinical response to adalimumab: relationship to anti-adalimumab antibodies and serum adalimumab concentrations in rheumatoid arthritis. Ann Rheum Dis. 2007;66:921–6.
18. Emery P, Gottenberg JE, Rubbert-Roth A, Sarzi-Puttini P, Choquette D, Martínez Taboada VM et al. Rituximab versus an alternative TNF inhibitor in patients with rheumatoid arthritis who failed to respond to a single previous TNF inhibitor: SWITCH-RA, a global, observational, comparative effectiveness study. Ann Rheum Dis. 2014; [Epub ahead of print].

Chapter 9
B-Cell Inhibition and Other Biologics

Abstract Most emphasis has been placed on the use of tumour necrosis factor inhibitors as the first line biologic agents in inflammatory arthritis patients not responding to DMARD therapy. There are, however, many other biological agents that are effective in DMARD-refractory individuals. Currently five other types of biologics are licensed for the management of inflammatory arthritis. Each drug inhibits a separate pathway involved in arthritis. These other biologics, viewed from the perspective of their mechanisms of action, comprise B-cell inhibition using Rituximab, T-cell modulation using Abatacept, interleukin-6 inhibition using Tocilizumab, interleukin-1 inhibition using Anakinra, and interleukin-12/-23 inhibition using Ustekinumab. This chapter will provide an overview of the mechanisms of action, clinical indications, side-effects and evidence base for each of these agents.

Keywords Biologics • Cytokines • Rituximab • Abatacept • Tocilizumab • Anakinra • Ustekinumab

Introduction

Although most emphasis has been placed on tumour necrosis factor inhibitors, there are many other biological agents that are effective in patients with inflammatory arthritis. Currently

I.C. Scott et al., *Inflammatory Arthritis in Clinical Practice*, 137
DOI 10.1007/978-1-4471-6648-1_9,
© Springer-Verlag London 2015

five other types of biologics are licensed for the management of inflammatory arthritis. Each drug inhibits a separate pathway involved in arthritis.

Two of these biologics affect cellular pathways, which involve either B-cells or T-cells. Three of them inhibit different cytokines. Four are effective in RA and one is effective in PsA. These other biologics, viewed from the perspective of their mechanisms of action, comprise:

- *B-cell inhibition:* Rituximab, which is effective in RA and is given by intravenous infusions.
- *T-cell modulation:* Abatacept, which is effective in RA and can be given by either intravenous infusion or subcutaneous injections.
- *Interleukin-6 (Il-6) inhibition:* Tocilizumab, which is effective in RA and can be given by either intravenous infusion or subcutaneous injections.
- *Interleukin-1 (Il-1) receptor antagonist:* Anakinra, which can be given in RA but has insufficient efficacy to justify its widespread use. Interestingly it is more effective in acute gout and a range of rarer disorders including familial fevers.
- *Interleukin-12/-23 (Il-12/-23) antagonist-* Ustekinumab

Rituximab

Background

Rituximab is a chimeric monoclonal antibody. It depletes the B-cell population by targeting cells bearing the CD20 surface marker [1]. This binding interferes with the activation and differentiation of B cells. It was introduced for the treatment of lymphomas but was subsequently found to be effective in RA. The effect on B-cells suggests that the prevailing view of RA as a predominantly T-cell mediated disease is doubtful.

B Cells in RA

The mechanism or mechanisms by which B cell depletion improves RA are unclear [2]. B cells have potentially important roles in several aspects of RA pathogenesis. Firstly they may act as antigen-presenting cells providing co-stimulatory signals for T cell activation and expansion. Secondly they are involved in the production of rheumatoid factor and anti-cyclic citrullinated peptide antibodies, which lead to immune complex formation and complement activation. These autoantibodies are associated with more severe disease phenotypes. Finally they can be involved in the production of pro-inflammatory cytokines such as TNF and IL-6. These cytokines drive the chronic inflammatory process which characterise active RA.

Mechanism of Action

Rituximab can deplete C20+ B cells by several mechanisms. These include inducing CD20+ B cell lysis by recruiting components of the innate immune system such as macrophages, inducing apoptosis of CD20+ B cells and activating the complement cascade leading to the formation of membrane attack complexes that target CD20+ B cells [2].

Clinical Indications

Rituximab is given in combination with methotrexate to treat severely active RA. Its use is currently focussed on patients who have had an inadequate response or intolerance to standard DMARDs and to one TNF-inhibitor.

Clinical Efficacy

A number of clinical trials have been completed, which all show rituximab reduces joint counts, improves disability and limits joint damage in patients with active RA. It is effective in both treatment naive patients and those refractory to previous DMARDs and TNF-inhibitors. Its use, however, is currently restricted to those with active RA who have failed anti-TNF treatment.

One systematic review has combined findings from three trials, which enrolled 938 patients with active RA [3]. They

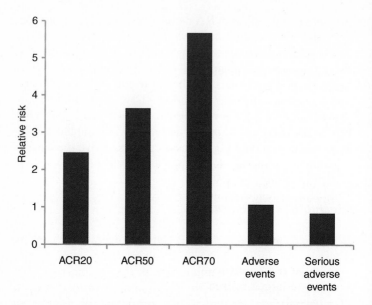

FIGURE 9.1 Effect of rituximab in active RA patients compared to methotrexate treated controls (Based on systematic review by Lee et al. [3]. Figure adapted using data reported by Lee et al. [3])

were all resistant or intolerant to DMARDs or TNF-inhibitors. They were followed up for 6–12 months. Patients receiving rituximab and methotrexate had substantially greater ACR responder rates without more toxicity. These results are summarised in Fig. 9.1

Although it is used in seropositive and seronegative RA patients, the efficacy of rituximab appears to be superior in seropositive individuals. A meta-analysis of four clinical trials identified modest but important clinical benefits in patients who are seropositive for rheumatoid factor and also for anti-cyclic citrullinated peptide antibodies [4]. The reduction at 6 months in DAS28 scores was 0.35 units higher in seropositive patients. The effects of rituximab also mirror rheumatoid factor levels. Serum autoantibody levels fall in association with clinical responses.

Initial and Repeat Courses

A course of rituximab comprises two 1 g intravenous infusions 2 weeks apart given alongside intravenous methylprednisolone. It is given with methotrexate, which potentiates its efficacy and durability. A single course of treatment results in a near total peripheral blood B cell population depletion. This usually persists for 6–9 months. CD20 is expressed on only pre-B cells and mature B cells; it is not expressed on stem cells or plasma cells. Therefore B cell repopulation occurs after this time point by naive B cells.

In patients who respond further infusions can be given at intervals of at least 6 months. The optimal time to give repeated infusions is not certain. Currently practiced regimens comprise:

1. Regular re-treatment: every 6-months
2. Treat-to-target: re-treat every 6 months until remission is achieved
3. Re-treatment on flare: an approach undertaken in early clinical trials

Although trial data indicates a treatment-to-target strategy may be best, limited long-term safety data in RA indicates the need for caution with regular re-treatment.

Adverse Reactions

Most adverse effects are infusion-related reactions, and are generally mild to moderate. Reactions to the first infusion such as hypotension and fever are common, occurring in one third of patients. They are reduced by corticosteroid prophylaxis with intravenous methylprednisolone. Such reactions are usually reversed by reducing or interrupting the infusion alongside therapeutic intervention with paracetamol and antihistamines. They are less common with repeated courses. Severe infusion reactions leading to drug discontinuation are rare occurring in less than one percent of patients.

A range of other adverse events may occur [5], and these have been studied in a cohort of 3,194 RA patients who had received up to 17 rituximab courses over 9.5 years. Rituximab remained well tolerated over time and multiple courses. There was no indication of an increased safety risk with rituximab over time.

Infection

There is a slightly increased rate of infection in RA patients receiving rituximab. Data from the biologics registries indicates that serious infections are greatest in the first few months following treatment. As with all biologics rituximab should be avoided in patients with an active infection or those who are severely immunocompromised.

Unlike anti-TNF therapy the risk of TB does not appear increased and there is no current evidence indicating the need to screen RA patients for TB prior to rituximab treatment.

Hepatitis B virus reactivation has been well documented in oncology patients, but not RA patients treated with rituximab. In patients with serological evidence of previous or current hepatitis B infection the risk-benefit profile should be fully discussed. If rituximab is deemed necessary then patient management should be undertaken in consultation with a gastroenterologist. Prophylactic treatment against hepatitis B reactivation with lamivudine may be considered. Current practice is to pre-screen patients for previous/current hepatitis B infection. The risk of hepatitis C virus is unclear although there are reports of severe infusion reactions in hepatitis C infected patients. It is recommended that patients should be screened for risk factors for hepatitis C pre-treatment.

To date a few cases of progressive multifocal leukoencephalopathy have been reported in RA patients. Most had long-standing RA with previous use of multiple immunosuppressive agents. Progressive multifocal leukoencephalopathy is caused by reactivation of the common JC virus. It occurs in immunocompromised individuals, resulting in myelin loss within the nervous system. Symptoms are protean and depend upon the location and degree of myelin loss. They include personality changes, visual disturbances and weakness. Although the risk is very small (currently estimated at 1 in 20,000) its poor prognosis and lack of specific treatment means that patients should receive pre-treatment counselling regarding it.

Anti-biologic Antibodies

Human anti-chimeric antibodies are detected in about 10 % of patients and may be associated with worse infusion or allergic reactions and failure to deplete B-cells after subsequent courses.

Tocilizumab

Background

IL-6 is an important pro-inflammatory cytokine in RA. It promotes inflammation through the expansion and activation of T cells, differentiation of B cells and induction of acute-phase reactants by hepatocytes. IL-6 signal transduction is mediated by membrane-bound and soluble receptors [6]. Tocilizumab is at present the only available IL-6 inhibitor for the treatment of inflammatory arthritis. It is a recombinant humanised anti-human IL-6 receptor monoclonal antibody of the IgG1 subclass. It binds to both membrane-bound and soluble IL-6 receptors, preventing their activation by IL-6.

Clinical Use

Tocilizumab is mainly used in patients with active RA who have failed treatment with standard DMARDs. It is usually given in combination with methotrexate. However it can be given as a monotherapy without methotrexate.

Dosing

The first approach to treatment was intravenously dosing adjusted for body weight given every 4 weeks. Dosing can be adjusted for problems such as deranged liver function tests, neutropenia or thrombocytopenia. More recently it has become available as weekly subcutaneous injections which are self-administered by patients. These are likely to become the most widely used treatment modality with tocilizumab.

Clinical Efficacy

Several systematic reviews have assessed the effectiveness of tocilizumab in RA. One review described experience in eight clinical trials involving 3,334 patients [7]. The other described experience in 12 trials involving 5,894 patients [8]. Their conclusions are similar. They show that tocilizumab increased the number of patients achieving ACR50 responses, and other ACR responses, there were more remissions with tocilizumab, including DAS28 remissions, and more patients achieved clinically important reductions in disability. These benefits are shown in Fig. 9.2.

Tocilizumab is beneficial in patients who have failed to respond to methotrexate and to tumour necrosis factor inhibitors. Although it is usually given with methotrexate, tocilizumab is also effective as monotherapy. Most research has focussed on using intravenous infusions of tocilizumab. However, it is now available for subcutaneous administration and is also effective when given by this route [9].

Adverse Events

The overall safety profile of Tocilizumab is acceptable. Most adverse events are mild to moderate in severity. Common adverse events with tocilizumab include infection, often nasopharyngitis, followed by gastrointestinal disturbance, stomatitis, rash, and headache.

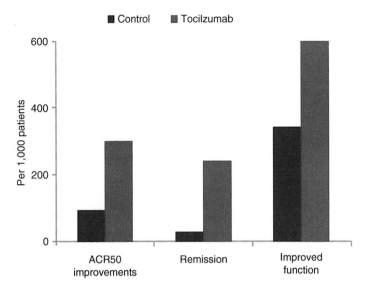

FIGURE 9.2 Key benefit of tocilizumab in clinical trials (Based on systematic review by Singh et al. [7]. Figure adapted using data reported by Singh et al. [7])

Infusion and Hypersensitivity Reactions

Infusion reactions may occur when intravenous tocilizumab is used. They include hypertension, which is usually seen during the infusion, headache, pruritis or rash. Hypersensitivity reactions are very rare.

Infection

As with all biologics the risk of infection is slightly increased. The incidence of serious infections is low; the most commonly reported comprising pneumonia and cellulitis. The risk of tuberculosis also appears to be increased. Current guidance recommends that as with TNF inhibitors patients should be screened for tuberculosis and those with latent infection administered chemoprophylaxis prior to treatment initiation.

Liver Function Test Abnormalities

Abnormalities of liver function tests are common in patients receiving tocilizumab, particularly in patients also receiving methotrexate. Most resolve spontaneously or with treatment modification such as dose reduction.

Elevated Lipids

Lipid elevations are commonly seen with up to one quarter of patients in clinical trials experiencing significant sustained total cholesterol elevations. These changes generally occur around treatment initiation and stabilise with time. Their impact on cardiovascular risk is unclear as high-density lipo-protein also increases with treatment and reducing systemic inflammation has a beneficial effect on atherogenesis. Current guidance recommends that standard guidelines for lipid management should be followed.

Neutropenia and Thrombocytopenia

IL-6 plays an important role in the recruitment of neutrophils from bone marrow stores into the peripheral blood. Tocilizumab thus results in an immediate but short-lived, dose dependent neutropenia. Serious neutropenia is uncommon. There is no clear relationship between neutropenia and serious infections. Blood count monitoring is recommended and neutropenia may be managed by a dose reduction. Thrombocytopenia has been reported but is less common than neutropenia. It is not associated with an increased bleeding risk. As with neutropenia a dose reduction may be necessary.

Anti-biologic Antibodies

Antibodies to tocilizumab can occur. They are rarer than with anti-TNF agents. Their precise clinical relevance is unknown.

Abatacept

Background

T cells, in particular CD4+ T cells, have well established roles in RA pathogenesis. T cells require two stimulatory signals to become activated. The primarily stimulatory signal is generated from the binding of the T cell receptor to MHC complexes containing a relevant antigen. The secondary co-stimulatory signal involves the binding of CD28 on the T cell to CD80 or CD86 on the antigen presenting cell.

Abatacept is a fusion protein comprising an immunoglobulin fused to the extracellular domain of cytotoxic T-lymphocyte antigen 4 (CTLA-4). CTLA-4 is a molecule that binds with a high affinity to the CD80/86 ligand on antigen presenting cells. The abatacept molecule therefore blocks the interaction between the CD80/86 ligand on the antigen presenting cell and the CD28 ligand on the T cell, preventing T cell activation. This results in reduced T-cell proliferation and cytokine production. T cell inhibition is a less focused form of immune modulating therapy than specific anti-cytokine agents; it results in a reduction of the cytokines TNF-α, IL-1 and IL-6. It also has implications on B cell activation.

Clinical Use

Abatacept, in combination with methotrexate, is used in patients with severely active RA who have responded inadequately to disease-modifying anti-rheumatic drugs including methotrexate.

Dosing

Abatacept was initially only available as an intravenous infusion. The exact dose depends on patient's weight. Maintenance intravenous dosing is needed every 4 weeks. More recently subcutaneous abatacept has become available [10] and this is given weekly. It is likely to be the main way of giving abatacept.

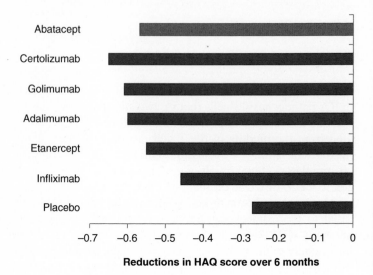

FIGURE 9.3 Comparable reductions in disability over 6 months with abatacept and other biologics (Based on systematic review by Maxwell and Singh [11]. Figure adapted using data reported by Maxwell and Singh [11])

Clinical Efficacy

Abatacept reduces disease activity, improves function and reduces erosive damage. Long-term extension data from clinical trials shows it retains effectiveness and protects against erosions for 5 years or longer.

An initial systematic review combined results from seven trials that involved 2,908 patients with RA [11]. It confirmed the overall clinical efficacy of abatacept and showed five patients needed to be treated to achieve an ACR50 response. A subsequent systematic review compared it with other biologics, showing broadly comparable benefits to TNF inhibitors [12]. An example of abatacept's effect on functional improvement is shown in Fig. 9.3

Adverse Reactions

There is extensive safety data for abatacept based on trials and observational studies of over 4,500 patients treated for over 12,000 years [13]. Infections are the main safety risk but their frequency does not increase over time. Overall the safety profile of abatacept is reassuring with low rates of serious adverse events. Minor problems like headache and nausea are common. Other frequent reactions include hypertension, rashes and fatigue. There is no evidence of an increased risk of malignancy.

Ustekinumab

Background

PsA involves different inflammatory pathways to RA. IL-17 is a key inflammatory cytokine produced by Th17 cells in response to IL-23. It is involved in the pathogenesis of PsA. Ustekinumab is a novel monoclonal antibody which targets the shared p40 subunit of IL12 and IL23. It is effective in both psoriasis and PsA [14].

Clinical Use

Ustekinumab is given by subcutaneous injection. After an initial dose, and a second dose after 4 weeks, it is given every 12 weeks. Clinical trials show that in PsA it gives greater 6 month ACR responses than placebo. It also reduces enthesitis and dactylitis scores, X-ray progression and disability scores. Responses are maintained during long-term therapy both with and without methotrexate [15]. At present many health services do not recommend using Ustekinumab routinely as the evidence for its cost-effectiveness is incomplete. This is likely to change with time.

Adverse Events

At present there is limited safety data on ustekinumab in PsA due to its relatively recent introduction as a treatment. However, there is more extensive information from its use in psoriasis [16]. There are concerns about risks from infection, malignancy and laboratory test abnormalities and hypersensitivity. So far there appear to be no major increased risks of these side-effects, but caution is needed.

Anakinra

Background

Interleukin-1β is an important cytokine in RA. It is produced excessively by the peripheral blood monocytes of RA patients when compared with healthy individuals. One IL-1 blocking agent, Anakinra, can be used to treat inflammatory arthritis. Anakinra is a recombinant human IL-1 receptor antagonist that inhibits the action of IL-1 by competitively blocking it's binding to IL-1 receptors on target cells. Its half-life after subcutaneous injection is 3–6 h.

Clinical Use

Trials have shown that anakinra improves active RA. However, its impact is relatively modest, even when given with methotrexate. It is therefore rarely used for RA, though it is approved for use in active disease.

More recently there has been an increasing appreciation of the role that Anakinra plays in the treatment of auto-inflammatory syndromes. Auto-inflammatory disorders are characterised by episodes of inflammation apparently involving unprovoked activation of the innate immune system. Examples of these diseases include Familial Mediterranean fever (FMF) and TNF-receptor associated periodic syndrome

(TRAPS). Although a clinically heterogeneous group of disorders, dysregulation of the IL-1 pathway appears to be pivotal in their pathogenesis. Their underlying causation appears to be abnormal activation of the inflammasome, an intracellular complex that on detection of foreign pathogens by pathogen-recognition receptors results in activation of IL-1β. Numerous case reports and series of exist outlining the successful treatment of these disorders with Anakinra [17].

Anakinra has also been shown to be an effective treatment for acute gout [18], with monosodium urate crystals causing pain and joint inflammation through the inflammasome with subsequent IL-1β activation. Due to its expense and the efficacy of NSAIDs, colchicine and corticosteroids in the management of acute gout it is not routinely used to treat this condition.

Side-Effects

Anakinra causes frequent injection site reactions, which may affect up to two thirds of patients; they do not usually require treatment. There is a small increased risk of infections, including serious infections. Anakinra should not be started and should be discontinued when these are present. There is no evidence that it increases the risk of tuberculosis and screening for this prior to treatment initiation is not required.

References

1. Tsokos GC. B cells, be gone–B-cell depletion in the treatment of rheumatoid arthritis. N Engl J Med. 2004;350:2546–8.
2. Shaw T, Quan J, Totoritis MC. B cell therapy for rheumatoid arthritis: the rituximab (anti-CD20) experience. Ann Rheum Dis. 2003;62 Suppl 2: ii55–9.
3. Lee YH, Bae SC, Song GG. The efficacy and safety of rituximab for the treatment of active rheumatoid arthritis: a systematic review and meta-analysis of randomized controlled trials. Rheumatol Int. 2011;31:1493–9.

4. Isaacs JD, Cohen SB, Emery P, Tak PP, Wang J, Lei G, et al. Effect of baseline rheumatoid factor and anticitrullinated peptide antibody serotype on rituximab clinical response: a meta-analysis. Ann Rheum Dis. 2013;72:329–36.

5. van Vollenhoven RF, Emery P, Bingham 3rd CO, Keystone EC, Fleischmann RM, Furst DE, et al. Long-term safety of rituximab in rheumatoid arthritis: 9.5-year follow-up of the global clinical trial programme with a focus on adverse events of interest in RA patients. Ann Rheum Dis. 2013;72:1496–502.

6. Dhillon S. Intravenous tocilizumab: a review of its use in adults with rheumatoid arthritis. BioDrugs. 2014;28:75–106.

7. Singh JA, Beg S, Lopez-Olivo MA. Tocilizumab for rheumatoid arthritis: a Cochrane systematic review. J Rheumatol. 2011;38:10–20.

8. Al-Shakarchi I, Gullick NJ, Scott DL. Current perspectives on tocilizumab for the treatment of rheumatoid arthritis: a review. Patient Prefer Adherence. 2013;7:653–66.

9. Burmester GR, Rubbert-Roth A, Cantagrel A, Hall S, Leszczynski P, Feldman D, et al. A randomised, double-blind, parallel-group study of the safety and efficacy of subcutaneous tocilizumab versus intravenous tocilizumab in combination with traditional disease-modifying antirheumatic drugs in patients with moderate to severe rheumatoid arthritis (SUMMACTA study). Ann Rheum Dis. 2014;73:69–74.

10. Genovese MC, Tena CP, Covarrubias A, Leon G, Mysler E, Keiserman M, et al. Subcutaneous abatacept for the treatment of rheumatoid arthritis: longterm data from the ACQUIRE trial. J Rheumatol. 2014;41:629–39.

11. Maxwell LJ, Singh JA. Abatacept for rheumatoid arthritis: a Cochrane systematic review. J Rheumatol. 2010;37:234–45.

12. Guyot P, Taylor PC, Christensen R, Pericleous L, Drost P, Eijgelshoven I, et al. Indirect treatment comparison of abatacept with methotrexate versus other biologic agents for active rheumatoid arthritis despite methotrexate therapy in the United kingdom. J Rheumatol. 2012;39:1198–206.

13. Atzeni F, Sarzi-Puttini P, Mutti A, Bugatti S, Cavagna L, Caporali R. Long-term safety of abatacept in patients with rheumatoid arthritis. Autoimmun Rev. 2013;12:1115–7.

14. Weitz JE, Ritchlin CT. Ustekinumab: targeting the IL-17 pathway to improve outcomes in psoriatic arthritis. Expert Opin Biol Ther. 2014;14:515–26.

15. McKeage K. Ustekinumab: a review of its use in psoriatic arthritis. Drugs. 2014;74:1029–39.

16. Papp KA, Griffiths CE, Gordon K, Lebwohl M, Szapary PO, Wasfi Y, et al. Long-term safety of ustekinumab in patients with moderate-to-severe psoriasis: final results from 5 years of follow-up. Br J Dermatol. 2013;168:844–54.
17. Akgul O, Kilic E, Kilic G, Ozgocmen S. Efficacy and safety of biologic treatments in Familial Mediterranean Fever. Am J Med Sci. 2013;346:137–41.
18. Ottaviani S, Molto A, Ea HK, Neveu S, Gill G, Brunier L, et al. Efficacy of anakinra in gouty arthritis: a retrospective study of 40 cases. Arthritis Res Ther. 2013;15:R123.

Chapter 10
Steroids

Abstract Steroids, in the form of glucocorticoids, are often used in the management of inflammatory arthritis patients. They exert anti-inflammatory and immunosuppressive effects via a range of different mechanisms, with the end-effect being a reduction in disease activity. They are often given intramuscularly in the form of methylprednisolone (depomedrone) during the early stages of arthritis when disease activity is high or during flares of the disease. Long-term low-dose oral steroids, in the form of prednisolone, are used, although this is becoming less common in the biologic era. Although often effective at reducing arthritis activity and preventing erosive progression, their use is restricted by their broad range of side-effects. In this chapter we will discuss the different types and methods of steroid administration in inflammatory arthritis patients, the evidence supporting their use and their side-effects.

Keywords Corticosteroids • Prednisolone • Depomederone • Local Injection • Side-Effects

Background

Steroids are given locally into joints or soft-tissues to treat synovitis, tenosynovitis and other local problems. They are given systemically as either high or low dose oral steroids by

I.C. Scott et al., *Inflammatory Arthritis in Clinical Practice*,
DOI 10.1007/978-1-4471-6648-1_10,
© Springer-Verlag London 2015

one or more intramuscular injections or by intravenous infusions. In each situation they have short-term efficacy. This benefit must be balanced against their long-term adverse events which can be serious. The clinical challenge is balancing their short-term benefits against their long-term risks [1].

The medical terminology is sometimes confusing. Using steroids to control inflammation involves exploiting their glucocorticoid properties. Many experts prefer to use the name glucocorticoids. Other steroids include mineralocorticoids, sex steroids and anabolic steroids. Nevertheless it is customary to use the generic term steroids when referring to glucocorticoids used to treat arthritis.

Pharmacological Effects

Steroids have complex anti-inflammatory and immunomodulatory effects. The term glucocorticoid reflects their involvement in glucose metabolism, which is a central effect of all glucocorticoids. Their anti-inflammatory and immunosuppressive effects involve a range of different mechanisms [2]. Steroids affect almost all immune cells. They inhibit white cell traffic and access to the sites of inflammation, interfere with the function of immune cells and suppress the production and actions of humoral factors. Many of their anti-inflammatory effects are mediated by cytosolic glucocorticoid receptors. These regulate proteins involved in inflammation and interfere with the function of transcription factors like nuclear factor-κB. Steroids also have rapid, nongenomic mechanisms, which are implicated in many of their immediate impacts.

In inflammatory arthritis steroids have impacts on the clinical symptoms of inflammation, which is partly due to infiltration of the synovium by lymphocytes. They also effect erosive progression, a process which is partly due to synovial infiltration by macrophages. Steroids influence the inflammatory process especially during the first months of treatment. They also have effects on erosions which are only evident after more prolonged treatment.

Steroids are metabolized in the liver. Consequently steroid effects are reduced by drugs that induce liver enzymes like phenytoin and rifampicin. Blood levels of steroids may rise in liver failure. Anticoagulant doses may need adjustment when given with steroids.

Cortisol, the classical glucocorticoid, is rarely used clinically. Synthetic glucocorticoids are preferred, which are more potent than cortisol. They differ in their pharmacokinetic properties, such as absorption and half-life, and the relative potency of their anti-inflammatory effects. Prednisolone is the dominant oral steroid and methylprednisolone (depomedrone) the dominant injectable steroid.

Effects on Joint Inflammation

Systemic steroids reduce joint inflammation in arthritis. They decrease the number of tender joints and swollen joints and reduce joint pain and elevated ESRs fall with treatment. A systematic review of the benefits of steroids report their benefits across 462 patients enrolled in 11 clinical trials [3]. The daily doses were 2.5–7.5 mg in four studies, 10 mg in three studies, and 15 mg in four. The low dose of steroids resulted in clinically significant improvements that lasted several months. Higher doses, such as 20 mg prednisolone daily, are also effective but are considered to have unacceptable risks of adverse effects.

Erosive Progression

There is extensive evidence that steroids reduce erosive damage, particularly in early arthritis when given in combination with disease modifying anti-rheumatic drugs. Even low dose steroids achieve this goal. A systematic review of the impact of steroids on erosive progression in RA included 1,414 patients enrolled in 15 trials [4]. All the trials except one showed treatment benefits in favour of steroids. The proportion of benefit from steroids in reducing the

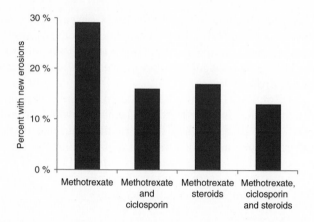

FIGURE 10.1 Reduction in new erosions by giving steroids with DMARDs in early rheumatoid arthritis (Figure produced using data from the Combination Anti-Rheumatic Drugs in Early RA (CARDERA) Trial [5])

progression of erosions from an average of all the studies over 1 year was 60 %. There is evidence for the steroids having a long-term benefit on erosive progression even if given for only 9 months or less. An example of the benefits of short-term steroids in early RA given with disease modifying drugs is shown in Fig. 10.1 [5].

Early Rheumatoid Arthritis

In early RA it is often thought there is a "window of opportunity" during which effective treatment can alter the course of the disease. There is strong evidence that steroids are particularly useful in these patients [6]. They have an immediate impact in reducing clinical symptoms of joint inflammation. They also reduce erosive damage. One drawback of using steroids in this way, apart from the risk of adverse effects, is that the effect on erosions may be small and short lived. The duration of the effect of steroids in this setting remains controversial.

Treating Flares with Systemic Steroids

Intramuscular steroid injections, particularly 120 mg methylprednisolone, help reduce flares. They also enhance the impact of starting DMARDs. Three to four monthly injections is helpful. Beyond that the evidence for continuing benefit is incomplete. On balance using intramuscular steroids for prolonged periods is counterproductive [7].

Intravenous steroids have been given and are rapidly effective. However, their use is often followed by a severe rebound in symptoms after 2–3 months. They are therefore not often used.

Psoriatic Arthritis and Ankylosing Spondylitis

Although many patients with PsA receive systemic steroids there is no evidence from clinical trials to support this approach [8]. There is some recent evidence in AS that they have short-term benefits [9]. However, the dose of steroids needed was relatively high, the benefits were short-term and the trial was relatively small. On balance, in patients with seronegative spondyloarthritis the benefits of systemic steroids remain uncertain, and their use should be limited and cautious.

Side-Effects

The disadvantages of systemic steroid use are their frequent and serious side-effects [10]. These problems, which are multiple, have been known for many years. Patients are concerned by general changes such as weight gain and oedema. Cardiovascular risks, especially accelerated atherosclerosis, are one major drawback. Other adverse events include hypertension, increased risk for diabetes and its complications, development of cataracts and increased incidence of glaucoma, increased susceptibility to infections, hyperlipidaemia, and gastrointestinal adverse events such as ulcers. Although many of these risks are dose-related, a large number of side effects can occur at relatively low doses.

Some adverse events are preventable, particularly osteoporosis. Systemic steroids increase the risk of fractures of the hip and spine. The greatest increase risk is seen with high-dose therapy. But increased risk is also seen at lower doses. Fracture risk increases rapidly after the onset of steroid treatment and declines equally rapidly after cessation of therapy. Loss of bone mineral density associated with oral steroids is therefore greatest in the first few months of their use. Patients at high risk of fracture, particularly those aged 65 years or over and those with a prior fragility fracture should commence bone-protective therapy at the time of starting steroids. In other individuals, measurement of bone mineral density using dual-energy X-ray absorptiometry (DEXA) is recommended for patients at risk.

Local Steroids

Steroid injections are used in individual joints to control local synovitis [11]. Patients show improvements in symptoms lasting a few weeks to a few months. This approach is more commonly used for large joints such as the knee.

Other sites that can be injected include entheses – where tendons are inserted into bones – and areas of compression, such as the carpal tunnel when there is median nerve compression.

Usually steroid injections are given without any imaging, but there is an increasing tendency to give steroids under ultrasound guidance. The evidence supporting this change is incomplete.

Injection of the sacroiliac joints may be beneficial for patients with seronegative arthritis, who have sacroiliac joint pain as part of a spondylo-arthropathy. This is best carried out under imaging control.

Adverse effects of local steroid injections are uncommon. Iatrogenic infection is potentially serious but rare. It occurs in less than one in 10,000 cases. More common, but less clinically important serious include local irritation, atrophy of soft tissues at the sites of injection and post-injection flares. There have been isolated reports of weakening and even rupture of tendons after local steroid use. Some patients suffer a loss of pigmentation, which can be permanent; this can be a problem for dark skinned individuals.

References

1. Bijlsma JW, Boers M, Saag KG, Furst DE. Glucocorticoids in the treatment of early and late RA. Ann Rheum Dis. 2003; 62:1033–7.
2. Spies CM, Bijlsma JW, Burmester GR, Buttgereit F. Pharmacology of glucocorticoids in rheumatoid arthritis. Curr Opin Pharmacol. 2010;10:302–7.
3. Gotzsche PC, Johansen HK. Short-term low-dose corticosteroids vs placebo and nonsteroidal antiinflammatory drugs in rheumatoid arthritis. Cochrane Database Syst Rev. 2005;(1):CD000189.
4. Kirwan JR, Bijlsma JW, Boers M, Shea BJ. Effects of glucocorticoids on radiological progression in rheumatoid arthritis. Cochrane Database Syst Rev. 2007;(1):CD006356.
5. Choy EH, Smith CM, Farewell V, Walker D, Hassell A, Chau L, et al. Factorial randomised controlled trial of glucocorticoids and combination disease modifying drugs in early rheumatoid arthritis. Ann Rheum Dis. 2008;67:656–63.
6. Gorter SL, Bijlsma JW, Cutolo M, Gomez-Reino J, Kouloumas M, Smolen JS, et al. Current evidence for the management of rheumatoid arthritis with glucocorticoids: a systematic literature review informing the EULAR recommendations for the management of rheumatoid arthritis. Ann Rheum Dis. 2010;69:1010–4.
7. Choy EH, Kingsley GH, Khoshaba B, Pipitone N, Scott DL, Intramuscular Methylprednisolone Study G. A two year randomised controlled trial of intramuscular depot steroids in patients with established rheumatoid arthritis who have shown an incomplete response to disease modifying antirheumatic drugs. Ann Rheum Dis. 2005;64:1288–93.
8. Fendler C, Baraliakos X, Braun J. Glucocorticoid treatment in spondyloarthritis. Clin Exp Rheumatol. 2011;29:S139–42.
9. Haibel H, Fendler C, Listing J, Callhoff J, Braun J, Sieper J. Efficacy of oral prednisolone in active ankylosing spondylitis:

results of a double-blind, randomised, placebo-controlled short-term trial. Ann Rheum Dis. 2014;73:243–6.

10. Kavanaugh A, Wells AF. Benefits and risks of low-dose glucocorticoid treatment in the patient with rheumatoid arthritis. Rheumatology (Oxford). 2014;53:1742–51.

11. Jacobs JW, Michels-van Amelsfort JM. How to perform local soft-tissue glucocorticoid injections? Best Pract Res Clin Rheumatol. 2013;27:171–94.

Chapter 11
Non-drug Treatments

Abstract   Treating inflammatory arthritis is not just a matter of giving medications. Patients require many non-drug approaches and treatments. These include education and advice, physiotherapy, occupational therapy, podiatry, psychological support and a range of orthopaedic interventions. This chapter will provide an overview of these crucial non-pharmacological management approaches.

Keywords   Patient Education • Physiotherapy • Occupational Therapy • Podiatry • Psychological Support

Background

Treating inflammatory arthritis is not just a matter of giving medications. Patients require many non-drug approaches and treatments. These include education and advice, physiotherapy, occupational therapy, podiatry, psychological support and a range of orthopaedic interventions.

Non-drug treatments can be considered in terms of which type of therapist is involved or by the overall aim of the treatment. This latter approach is preferable in that it does not specify that treatments should be given by one specific group of clinicians and that overlapping skills are needed.

I.C. Scott et al., *Inflammatory Arthritis in Clinical Practice*,
DOI 10.1007/978-1-4471-6648-1_11,
© Springer-Verlag London 2015

An overview of different non-drug therapies in RA [1] found 382 research studies dealing with approaches. They found the evidence was strongest for aerobic activities, dynamic muscular reinforcement and therapeutic patient education.

The situation is somewhat different in AS, where there is a greater emphasis on exercise for the spine [2]. An overview on non-drug therapies in these patients concluded that the cornerstone of non-pharmacological treatment is patient education and regular exercise. The experts involved also thought that home exercises are effective but that supervised exercises should be preferred. Finally in these patients self-help groups may be useful. In PsA the non-drug therapies needed often merge approaches used in RA and AS, depending on the particular problems in an individual patient.

Finally patients may use a variety of alternative medical approaches. Some of these focus on taking vitamins and other supplementary treatments, some involve systems of medicine such as homeopathy, and many involve dietary changes. Though these alternative approaches are favoured by many patients, there is very little evidence that they are effective.

Multidisciplinary Teams

Patients with inflammatory arthritis should be treated by a multidisciplinary team rather than by an individual clinician. The exact make-up of the team will differ between units depending on a range of local circumstances [3]. Key members of the team include rheumatologists, specialist nurses, physiotherapists, occupational therapists and podiatrists. Patients are often involved in making decisions about the care they receive and therefore may sometimes be considered part of the team. Ideally primary care clinicians and surgeons would also be involved. Although many clinicians are involved in the team, one member needs to have overall responsibility for coordinating care between the various health professionals involved. Often this role will be taken by a specialist nurse.

Education and Support

The diagnosis of inflammatory arthritis has a negative impact on patients. They need support and advice to deal with their anxieties about their condition and its management. Most often this is provided by rheumatology specialist nurses. Education can be provided for individual patients or groups of patients. The approach chosen reflects patient preferences and local custom and practice. It is also possible to incorporate education within clinic visits by providing structured support from clinicians; one example of this approach is collaborative goal-setting with patients. An expert review of the area [4] highlighted that information is a prerequisite to education and that appropriate education can empower patients to take an active part in managing their disease. It will also improve coping and enhance adherence with treatment regimens.

Promoting Coping

It is essential to help patients deal with their arthritis. A range of approaches can be used. These include promoting self-management approaches and attempting to instil a readiness to change. Cognitive-behavioural approaches, which can be employed by a range of clinicians, can help promote health behaviour change. Other psychological therapies may also be useful. These include relaxation training and stress and mood management as well as formal cognitive behavioural therapy. Promoting coping can usually be combined with patient education and exercise programmes [5].

Promoting Mobility, Function and Participation

Equally important is to promote mobility and enhance function. This can be achieved in several ways. Supportive information can underline the benefits of exercise and joint protection and promote lifestyle physical activity. Historically clinicians advised patients with arthritis to rest. This approach has now been reversed. Patients should be given advice and training to improve general and musculoskeletal fitness. Examples include individualised walking and fitness programmes and group or individual joint protection training, which include hand exercises and fatigue management.

General advice should be supported by specific therapy to help individual needs. Physiotherapy can help by providing exercise programmes, balance training, hydrotherapy and mobility aids. Occupational therapy can help by providing work advice and rehabilitation, training for activities of daily living, environmental modifications, orthoses, a range of social and leisure rehabilitation methods and some psychological therapies. Finally, podiatry can help by giving foot care and footwear advice, foot orthoses and custom shoes.

Physiotherapy

Physiotherapy uses a range of physical approaches with the aim of reducing pain, preventing deformity and maximising function. These aims are achieved by using a range of interventions. Some are active interventions and others are more passive (Table 11.1).

A number of guidelines for physiotherapy in inflammatory arthritis exist and these have been evaluated by an expert group [6]. They found that recommendations on exercise therapy and patient education were included in all guidelines. Other treatment modalities including transcutaneous nerve stimulation and thermotherapy were recommended in most but not all guidelines and a few treatment approaches such as ultrasound were only recommended occasionally. Recommendations on physiotherapy interventions were variable and often, lacked detail concerning mode of delivery, intensity, frequency and duration.

Educating patients about what they can do to improve their arthritis and exercise to maintain function are key issues. Until recently there were concerns that exercise would

TABLE 11.1 Range of physiotherapy treatments

Treatment modality	Examples
Patient education and self-management	Joint protection methods
	Pain relief strategies
	Relaxation training
	Exercise and physical activity recommendations
Exercise therapy	Aerobic activities
	Muscle strengthening
	Core stability exercise
	Balance rehabilitation
	Hydrotherapy
Manual therapy	Mobilisation and manipulation
	Myofascial release and trigger point therapy
	Acupuncture
Thermotherapy	Heat and cold to reduce inflammatory pain
Electro-physical agents	Transcutaneous Electrical Nerve Stimulation (TENS)
	Ultrasound
	Pulsed Electromagnetic Energy (PEME)
	Interferential therapy (IFT)
	Laser
Assistive devices	Walking aids
	Splints
	Orthoses

accelerate joint damage. However, this has not proved to be the case and there is now greater emphasis on dynamic conditioning exercise. Strategies for exercise are designed to improve health-related fitness without exacerbating joint damage. The benefits of physical activity requires regular and sustained exercise, and adherence with the planned treatment is essential.

Passive treatments depend less on patient concordance but are less likely to provide an overall benefit. The range spans manual therapy techniques and electrophysical approaches such as heat and cold. These are used to solve specific clinical problems for short periods of time. Other methods include manual therapy, electrophysical agents such as Transcutaneous Electrical Nerve Stimulation (TENS) and ultrasound, and providing assistive devices like walking sticks.

Although a wide range of physical treatments can be used the best evidence for efficacy is for exercise. This has both physical and psychological benefits. Aerobic exercise programmes improve of fitness, improve psychological status, reduce pain and enhance function without exacerbating disease activity or accelerating joint damage. Overall it is more effective to provide a comprehensive package of care in a community setting addressing the needs of specific patients by education, exercise and pain relief modalities.

In AS the emphasis is on exercise, which is the most studied physiotherapy modality [7]. There is strong support for exercise in these patients and it can be delivered in a variety of ways. Exercise improves pain, spinal mobility, function, fatigue and quality of life.

Occupational Therapy

The goal of occupational therapy is improving patients abilities to perform daily activities and participate in life activities at work, in the home and socially. In addition therapists help adapt lifestyles and minimise functional and psychological problems. Comprehensive programmes include a wide range of interventions. Occupational therapists are trained in both

TABLE 11.2 Range of occupational therapy treatments

Treatment modality	Examples
Joint protection	Maintaining function through altering working methods
	Education in joint and body mechanics
Assistive devices	Hand (e.g. jar openers and ergonomic vegetable peelers), Knee and hip (e.g. aids and toilet raisers)
	Reduced mobility (e.g. half-steps and stair rails)
Splinting	Resting splints
	Working splints
Hand therapy	Use of joint protection and splinting for hands
Work rehabilitation	On-site assessments
	Ergonometric adaptations
Comprehensive (additional components)	Stress and pain management
	Relaxation training
	Counselling

physical and mental health rehabilitation. They are therefore able to help people with arthritis cope with the problems of multiple functional difficulties, pain, stress and low mood.

A range of different treatment approaches exist (Table 11.2). They have not all been fully evaluated. When experts have considered all the available evidence they concluded there was only limited evidence for the effectiveness of occupational therapy for functional ability and pain [8]. There was also some evidence that comprehensive occupational therapy and instruction on joint protection improved functional ability. However, it is challenging to undertake definitive research in this complex area. Nevertheless the balance of evidence suggests a comprehensive programme of occupational therapy is likely to improve patients' ability to cope with arthritis and should be provided early in the course of the disease.

Podiatry

Feet are commonly involved in inflammatory arthritis. Involvement of the joints of the feet causes reduced mobility and impaired function. In about three quarters of people with inflammatory arthritis of the feet contributes to difficulty with walking; it is the main problem in many people. Regrettably the area is relatively overlooked.

Podiatrists can help people with arthritis in four main ways. Firstly they can provide education about foot problems and give advice on footwear. Secondly, they can help provide orthoses and footwear. Thirdly they can arrange general foot care, which will include support with nail cutting, corn and callus reduction and providing padding. Finally in patients with risks of vasculitic or ulcerative foot involvement they can provide help in reducing the risks of progression. The evidence for benefit is strongest with insoles and footwear [9].

Orthopaedic Surgery

The surgical treatment of arthritis is a subject in its own right. It is impractical to provide detailed guidance on this complex area in a short book on medical treatments. At the same time it is inappropriate to entirely ignore this important issue for many patients. It is also an area in which there have been dramatic changes in approach [10].

The most important contribution of surgery is the replacement of failed joints. The knee and hip are the most important examples, but shoulder and elbow replacements are also important. Equally effective is the prevention of damage to tendons by timely intervention to prevent rupture or to repair ruptured tendons at an early stage. Finally a small minority of patients have major problems with their cervical spine and may require surgical intervention to prevent cord damage.

Patients should be referred for review by an orthopaedic surgeon if they have:

(a) Persistent pain resulting from joint damage or soft tissue involvement
(b) Declining function
(c) Increasing deformity
(d) Continuing localised synovitis

There are a number of other reasons such as potential or definite tendon rupture, nerve compression, joint instability, joint infection and stress fractures. Multiple tendon rupture, persisting neurological deficit and non-correctable deformity causing disability should be avoided by early referral in patients at risk of these problems.

References

1. Forestier R, Andre-Vert J, Guillez P, Coudeyre E, Lefevre-Colau MM, Combe B, et al. Non-drug treatment (excluding surgery) in rheumatoid arthritis: clinical practice guidelines. Joint Bone Spine. 2009;76:691–8.
2. Braun J, van den Berg R, Baraliakos X, Boehm H, Burgos-Vargas R, Collantes-Estevez E, et al. 2010 update of the ASAS/EULAR recommendations for the management of ankylosing spondylitis. Ann Rheum Dis. 2011;70:896–904.
3. Vliet Vlieland TP. Multidisciplinary team care and outcomes in rheumatoid arthritis. Curr Opin Rheumatol. 2004;16:153–6.
4. Fautrel B, Pham T, Gossec L, Combe B, Flipo RM, Goupille P, et al. Role and modalities of information and education in the management of patients with rheumatoid arthritis: development of recommendations for clinical practice based on published evidence and expert opinion. Joint Bone Spine. 2005;72:163–70.
5. Manning VL, Hurley MV, Scott DL, Coker B, Choy E, Bearne LM. Education, self-management, and upper extremity exercise training in people with rheumatoid arthritis: a randomized controlled trial. Arthritis Care Res. 2014;66:217–27.
6. Hurkmans EJ, Jones A, Li LC, Vliet Vlieland TP. Quality appraisal of clinical practice guidelines on the use of physiotherapy in rheumatoid arthritis: a systematic review. Rheumatology (Oxford). 2011;50:1879–88.

7. Passalent LA. Physiotherapy for ankylosing spondylitis: evidence and application. Curr Opin Rheumatol. 2011;23:142–7.

8. Steultjens EM, Dekker J, Bouter LM, van Schaardenburg D, van Kuyk MA, van den Ende CH. Occupational therapy for rheumatoid arthritis: a systematic review. Arthritis Rheum. 2002;47:672–85.

9. Hennessy K, Woodburn J, Steultjens MP. Custom foot orthoses for rheumatoid arthritis: a systematic review. Arthritis Care Res. 2012;64:311–20.

10. Nikiphorou E, Konan S, MacGregor AJ, Haddad FS, Young A. The surgical treatment of rheumatoid arthritis: a new era? Bone Joint J. 2014;96-B:1287–9.

Chapter 12
Stopping Treatments

Abstract Inflammatory arthritis is often a long-term condition that can persist for decades. Treatment is usually continued long-term, increasing the exposure of patients to potential adverse events. Although stopping treatment entirely once a patient's disease activity is well controlled is associated with a significantly increased risk of flaring, there is a growing body of evidence that it is possible to successfully taper DMARD, steroid and biologic treatments in patients who have achieved sustained remissions in their arthritis. This chapter provides an overview of withdrawing treatment in inflammatory arthritis patients, covering the possible approaches used and the evidence supporting them.

Keywords Treatment Tapering • Treatment Withdrawal • Step-Down Therapy • Disease Flare

Introduction

Inflammatory arthritis is usually a long-term condition. It can persist for years and decades. Two different decisions need to be made about the timing of treatment. The first decision is when to start treatment. The second decision is when to stop

I.C. Scott et al., *Inflammatory Arthritis in Clinical Practice*,
DOI 10.1007/978-1-4471-6648-1_12,
© Springer-Verlag London 2015

it. This chapter deals with the latter clinical problem. This problem is important as patients are often enthusiastic to have their treatment minimised [1].

Conventional Disease Modifying Drugs (DMARDs)

Can Patients Stay on DMARDs?

The first issue to consider is how long patients are able to remain on DMARDs, particularly if they continue to need them. Most patients who start DMARD monotherapy do not stay on treatment with single DMARDs indefinitely [2]. More than half the patients who start treatment with a single DMARD have had to stop treatment after 2–3 years. Retention rates differ across different DMARDs. Patients stay longer on methotrexate than other DMARDs. The probability of continuing methotrexate for 5 years approaches 80 %. For other DMARDs retention rates are lower. They may be no more than 30 % after 2 years treatment. Such low retention rates of patients starting DMARDs mean it is crucial to consider carefully the benefits and risks of discontinuing DMARDs in patients in whom therapy is controlling RA without causing adverse effects.

Withdrawing DMARDs in Responders

There have been many attempts to stop DMARDs when patients have achieved good clinical responses [3]. This has included a substantial number of clinical trials of treatment withdrawal. Most of these trials are historical. They mainly studied DMARD withdrawal in patients with RA who were in remission or were achieving good clinical responses. They followed patients for as long as 2 years. Most involved classical DMARDs such as gold and penicillamine, though these are not widely used today.

About one fifth of patients who continued to take DMARDs flared. In contrast about two fifth of patients who stopped DMARDs had a flare. When patients who had stopped DMARDs restarted treatment most regained control of their disease. Only a few patients did not benefit from resuming DMARDs.

Step-Down DMARD Therapy

One way to give intensive treatment is to start several DMARDs at the same time [4]. They can then be stepped down to DMARD monotherapy. This approach is particularly favoured in early RA. Several trials have evaluated using two conventional DMARDs, usually methotrexate and sulfasalazine, with prednisolone. Treatment is then stepped down after 6 months or longer to DMARD monotherapy. Patients benefit from the use of intensive treatment without the need to take combinations of drugs indefinitely. Overall trials in early and established RA show that step-down combination therapy is effective and has sustained benefits. Remaining on one anchor DMARD reduces subsequent flares. The optimal maintenance DMARD therapy has not been identified in these trials. However, most experts believe methotrexate is the best anchor drug to continue as monotherapy.

Observational Studies of DMARD Withdrawal

Several historical case series looked at reducing the frequency of DMARD administration [5]. Reducing methotrexate from weekly to fortnightly did not appear to cause more flares. The same was seen when reducing the frequency of giving penicillamine, though clearly the relevance of findings with this historical DMARD to current practice is uncertain.

There is some evidence that when patients are receiving biological treatment with infliximab the dose of methotrexate can be tapered without an increased risk of flares.

Despite these positive findings the long-term goal of "drug-free" remission remains elusive. It is only rarely achieved. About 10 % of patients in early arthritis cohorts who require DMARDs can eventually achieve sustained drug free remissions when treatments are stopped.

Predicting Flares After DMARD Withdrawal

Detailed analyses of early rheumatoid cohorts have identified several predictors of drug-free remissions [6]. These are symptom duration, rheumatoid factor positivity and presence of the *HLA-DRB1* shared epitope alleles. Rheumatoid factor positivity is the strongest predictor and seropositive patients are far less likely to be able to withdraw treatment than seronegative patients.

Recommendations in Guidelines

After reviewing the available evidence, expert groups have different perspectives about discontinuing DMARDs. There appears to be no overall consensus. UK guidelines from the National Institute for Health and Care Excellence (NICE) recommend that if RA is stable, DMARD doses should be cautiously reduced, returning promptly to disease controlling doses if there are any indications of a flare [7]. EULAR European guidelines are more guarded about DMARD tapering. They recommend that in sustained long-term remission cautious titration of synthetic DMARD dose may be considered [8]. By contrast American College of Rheumatology guidelines do not comment on DMARD withdrawal [9].

Biological Treatments

Stopping and Tapering

Most existing clinical research on tumour necrosis factor inhibitors in RA focuses on their efficacy and safety. The key driver of research has been to show tumour necrosis factor inhibitors and other biologics improve active inflammatory arthritis. An important question, which has received far less attention, is how to maintain response after disease control is achieved. By default doses of biologics effective in inducing responses in active arthritis have been continued to maintain control, though there is no evidence that continued high doses are needed

If disease control can be maintained with lower doses of biologics, the cost-effectiveness of these expensive treatments will increase. It should also lower the risks of serious adverse events. There are two approaches to decreasing treatment. One approach is to reduce the frequency of dosing, which means that treatment has been tapered. The other is to stop treatment completely. With the growing focus on intensive and rapid escalation of treatment in early active arthritis, it is particularly important that consideration is given to reducing the dosage of biologics when full control is achieved.

Studies in Rheumatoid Arthritis

A number of trials and observational studies have included an assessment of reducing the dose or stopping treatment with biologics in patients with inflammatory arthritis [10]. In virtually all these trials patients have continued to take DMARDs, particularly methotrexate. At the end of the early trials of infliximab in RA patients had their biologic stopped. Most of these patients flared, though control was regained when patients restarted treatment. Starting treatment again did not lead to an excess of adverse reactions.

When patients with RA have achieved sustained low disease activity or remission on biologics, particular tumour necrosis factor inhibitors, tapering treatment often maintains clinical response without the disease flaring. Stopping treatment entirely is more likely to lead to flares. However, in all studies, when treatment with biologics is restarted, disease control is re-established.

Studies in Psoriatic Arthritis

There is virtually no data on treatment tapering and stopping in PsA [11]. There is some evidence for observational studies that when patients have achieved remission treatment can be interrupted without major disadvantages. However, there have been no formal studies or trials on this theme.

Studies in Ankylosing Spondylitis

There is relatively little information about treatment tapering in AS patients. The information that is available suggests that in some patients who have achieved good clinical responses treatment intervals can be increased [12]. When patients stop treatment entirely they usually have a relapse after some months, though such relapses usually respond to restarting treatment.

Steroids

Intramuscular steroids and intra-articular steroids are invariably given intermittently. Their use is designed to ensure patients do not receive long-term treatment. Consequently, tapering and stopping are not relevant considerations.

Oral steroids bring short-term benefits. However, the overwhelming balance of evidence suggests in the long-term their use leads to more adverse events than benefits. As a consequence there is a strong rationale for stopping treatment.

In early arthritis most studies show that both short-term high dose and medium term intermediate dose steroids can be tapered and then stopped without major disadvantages. In established arthritis the evidence is incomplete [13].

When patients have taken steroids for prolonged periods of time treatment should gradually be tapered by about

1 mg per month [14]. Most patients can gradually reduce and stop treatment over 6–12 months or longer. Some patients flare and need short-term increases in steroid dosing. Despite the frequency of use of steroids and the need to minimise dosing, there is relatively limited research on steroid tapering. However, all expert groups agree that minimising and stopping steroids whenever possible is of critical importance.

Conclusions

There is nothing worse than agreeing to discontinue treatment in a patient with inflammatory arthritis who is in sustained clinical remission and then to discover over time that the disease flares and it is impossible to regain control. Most experienced clinicians will have come across this scenario at some time or other. It has a major and potentially disproportional impact on future practice.

Such an occasional negative occurrence must be weighed against the substantial weight of evidence that shows it is possible to successfully taper DMARD, steroid and biologic treatments in patients who have achieved sustained remissions in their arthritis. Stopping treatment completely seems less practical. When patients do stop treatment, it is usually possible to regain control by restarting treatment. Patients with RA may do better if they are left on a single DMARD. As DMARDs are relatively ineffective in AS, the likelihood of stopping biologic treatments in these patients seems less.

Leaving patients on long-term treatments that are over and above those needed to maintain disease control has two negative features. Firstly, it risks more adverse events. Secondly, it is unlikely to be cost-effective, and this latter point is particularly important with high cost biologic treatments. Therefore on balance when patients achieve sustained remission the best advice appears to be to taper and minimise but not entirely stop treatment.

References

1. Markusse IM, Akdemir G, Huizinga TW, Allaart CF. Drug-free holiday in patients with rheumatoid arthritis: a qualitative study to explore patients' opinion. Clin Rheumatol. 2014;33:1155–9.
2. Maetzel A, Wong A, Strand V, Tugwell P, Wells G, Bombardier C. Meta-analysis of treatment termination rates among rheumatoid arthritis patients receiving disease-modifying anti-rheumatic drugs. Rheumatology (Oxford). 2000;39:975–81.
3. Scott IC, Kingsley GH, Scott DL. Can we discontinue synthetic disease-modifying anti-rheumatic drugs in rheumatoid arthritis? Clin Exp Rheumatol. 2013;31:S4–8.
4. Boers M, van Tuyl L, van den Broek M, Kostense PJ, Allaart CF. Meta-analysis suggests that intensive non-biological combination therapy with step-down prednisolone (COBRA strategy) may also 'disconnect' disease activity and damage in rheumatoid arthritis. Ann Rheum Dis. 2013;72:406–9.
5. O'Mahony R, Richards A, Deighton C, Scott D. Withdrawal of disease-modifying antirheumatic drugs in patients with rheumatoid arthritis: a systematic review and meta-analysis. Ann Rheum Dis. 2010;69:1823–6.
6. van der Woude D, Young A, Jayakumar K, Mertens BJ, Toes RE, van der Heijde D, et al. Prevalence of and predictive factors for sustained disease-modifying antirheumatic drug-free remission in rheumatoid arthritis: results from two large early arthritis cohorts. Arthritis Rheum. 2009;60:2262–71.
7. National Institute for Health and Care Excellence. NICE technology appraisal guidance 130 adalimumab, etanercept and infliximab for the treatment of rheumatoid arthritis. 2007. http://www.nice.org.uk/guidance/ta130. Accessed 29 Oct 2014.
8. Smolen JS, Landewe R, Breedveld FC, Buch M, Burmester G, Dougados M, et al. EULAR recommendations for the management of rheumatoid arthritis with synthetic and biological disease-modifying antirheumatic drugs: 2013 update. Ann Rheum Dis. 2014;73:492–509.
9. Singh JA, Furst DE, Bharat A, Curtis JR, Kavanaugh AF, Kremer JM, et al. 2012 update of the 2008 American College of Rheumatology recommendations for the use of disease-modifying antirheumatic drugs and biologic agents in the treatment of rheumatoid arthritis. Arthritis Care Res. 2012;64: 625–39.

10. van Herwaarden N, den Broeder AA, Jacobs W, van der Maas A, Bijlsma JW, van Vollenhoven RF, et al. Down-titration and discontinuation strategies of tumor necrosis factor-blocking agents for rheumatoid arthritis in patients with low disease activity. Cochrane Database Syst Rev. 2014;(9):CD010455.

11. Moverley AR, Coates LC, Helliwell PS. Can biologic therapies be withdrawn or tapered in psoriatic arthritis? Clin Exp Rheumatol. 2013;31:S51–3.

12. Lee J, Noh JW, Hwang JW, Oh JM, Kim H, Ahn JK, et al. Extended dosing of etanercept 25 mg can be effective in patients with ankylosing spondylitis: a retrospective analysis. Clin Rheumatol. 2010;29:1149–54.

13. Boers M. The COBRA trial 20 years later. Clin Exp Rheumatol. 2011;29:S46–51.

14. Bacon PA, Myles AB, Beardwell CG, Daly JR. Corticosteroid withdrawal in rheumatoid arthritis. Lancet. 1966;2:935–7.

Chapter 13
Emerging Therapies in Rheumatoid Arthritis

Abstract The high costs of biologic agents, allied to the fact that not all patients will respond to them, means there is a major research focus on developing novel treatments for RA patients. One solution to these high costs is the development of "biosimilar" drugs. These are biological products that are highly similar to existing licensed biologics, allowing for minor differences in clinically inactive components, and for which there are no clinically meaningful differences in terms of product safety, purity, and potency. Another solution that would address both cost and non-responders is the development of small molecule agents, which target cellular structures and intracellular signalling proteins such as Janus Kinases. This chapter will provide an overview of the emerging therapeutic options for RA patients, spanning biosimilars, Janus Kinase inhibitors, other kinase inhibitors, PDE4 inhibitors and future potential therapeutic targets such as IL-17 inhibition.

Keywords Biosimilars • Small Molecule Drugs • Janus Kinase Inhibitors • Tofacitinib

I.C. Scott et al., *Inflammatory Arthritis in Clinical Practice*,
DOI 10.1007/978-1-4471-6648-1_13,
© Springer-Verlag London 2015

Introduction

The last decade has seen an unprecedented expansion in the therapeutic options available to treat RA. The growing number of effective biologic drugs highlights the complex nature of the human immune system. It has become apparent that similar clinical responses can be obtained by blocking any number of immune pathways. It therefore seems likely, given the enormous number of potential immunologic mechanisms at play in RA that many more therapeutic targets exist. The game change that biologics have brought about is the appreciation of the success of highly specific drugs.

However, biologic agents face several challenges: first, they are very expensive, and only marketed by a limited number of pharmaceutical companies; second, they are large proteins, which means they are both subject to immunogenicity and also are unable to be used to target intracellular immunologic pathways. The solutions to these problems are imminent.

Biosimilars

The pharmaceutical regulators define a biosimilar as a biological product that is "highly similar to an existing licensed biologic, allowing for minor differences in clinically inactive components, and for which there are no clinically meaningful differences between the biological product and the reference product in terms of the safety, purity, and potency of the product".

The concept of a biosimilar is not a new one, with such products available for drugs such as insulin or colony stimulating factors having been available for many years. The biologics used in rheumatic diseases differ from existing biosimilars though, being far more intricate entities, comprising large proteins with complex tertiary and quarternary structures that are challenging to duplicate. As such, it is not feasible to produce truly identical products, as subtle changes in structure, such as those that occur in post-translational modification, can never be entirely consistent: hence the use of the term 'biosimilar' rather than 'bioequivalent' [1]. Even small differences in compound structure can result in variation in clinical efficacy and safety. Therefore the regulatory authorities have imposed stringent requirements on manufacturers developing biosimilar agents to ensure that clinical (but not structural) equivalence is confirmed before marketing authorisation is approved [2]. It is also important to acknowledge that the potential differences in biosimilars to their reference compound will be within the range of variability that is currently observed with batch-to-batch variation of existing products [3].

Interchangeability of Biosimilars with Existing Agents

The European Regulators do not have the authority to enable automatic substitution of biosimilars with reference agents – this is a decision that will need making at a national level [1]. However, such a move would potentially enable pharmacists to switch agents without clinician assent. Such practice raises important concerns. It is known that with existing agents a key challenge is the development of anti-drug antibodies. Such immunogenicity is associated with adverse events and loss of efficacy [4]. In addition it is apparent that an important factor associated with immunogenicity is intermittent dosing regimens [5]. A theoretical concern is that intermittent dosing of an individual with a biosimilar agent and then a reference agent could have a similar effect upon immunogenicity. Therefore, until data are available, switching between products will not be recommended. A practical consideration following from this is that prescription of biologics should move to branded prescribing by clinicians.

However, it is clear that modern manufacturing techniques are superior to those available two decades ago when biologics first emerged in rheumatology and it would be wrong to assume that biosimilars will not perform as well as the reference compounds; evidence to date suggests they are as effective and in the future it is of course possible performance will exceed existing products. Crucially, the arrival of biosimilars will enact a substantial downwards shift in the price of biologics in rheumatology, which funding bodies urgently need.

Drugs in Development

The advent of biologic therapies has highlighted the importance of delivering drugs that have a specific target. However, biologics are also limited by a requirement for parenteral administration, an inability to enter cells and also the risk of immunogenicity. In recent years there has been a surge in the development of highly targeted small molecules that block pathways downstream of where the current biologics are acting. Such agents would be available orally, and not run the risk of immunogenicity.

JAK Inhibitors

The Janus Kinase (JAK) inhibitor class is already licensed in the US and at the time of writing is currently awaiting a decision from the regulators in Europe. The JAK inhibitors specifically bind and block members of the JAK enzyme family (JAK1, JAK2, JAK3 or TYK2). The resultant effect is to suppress the downstream production of inflammatory mediators. Under normal circumstances, JAK phosphorylates a transmembrane cytokine receptor in response to an extracellular signal (for example activation by IL-6). The signal is then transmitted to the nucleus of the cell via a number of routes including the Signal Transducer and Activator of Transcription (STAT) pathway. Subsequent nuclear effects result in increase production of new inflammatory proteins (including TNF). Therefore, given the knowledge of success in blocking both IL-6 and TNF pathways, JAK inhibition represents an obvious target in RA.

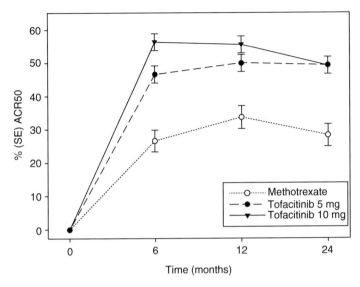

FIGURE 13.1 ACR50 response rates from a clinical trial of tofacitinib, an oral Janus Kinase inhibitor, versus methotrexate monotherapy in 958 RA patients. Significantly greater ACR50 response rates seen at all time-points with Tofacitinib therapy compared with methotrexate (P<0.001) (Figure adapted using data reported by Lee et al. [6])

Tofacitinib is a specific inhibitor of the JAK1 and JAK3 pathways and is the only currently licensed JAK inhibitor for rheumatoid at present. The phase 3 trial efficacy data showed superior efficacy of tofacitinib over methotrexate (Fig. 13.1) [6]. Across the breadth of publications regarding JAK inhibitors it seems clear that blocking JAK is an efficacious option (probably equivalent to many of the biologics), however there are limitations including important adverse effects. There is a risk of cytopenias (especially anaemia) and an increased rate of some infections including shingles in particular appears to be a concern. As more post-marketing safety data emerge the role of these agents in the treatment paradigm will become clearer.

Other Kinase Inhibitors

There are numerous other intracellular kinase pathways that have been investigated in RA. Bruton's tyrosine kinase (BTK) is a molecule that is central to B cell development and proliferation. Interest in B cells in RA has gained significant momentum since the success of rituximab. BTK inhibitors have also been developed and established in the treatment of B cell leukamias and so therapeutic agents are available. However, there is an important human model of BTK deficiency in children (Bruton's Agammaglobulinaemia) that results in a state of severe immunodeficiency characterised by antibody deficiency and recurrent infections. Therefore as this drug emerges into the rheumatology field there will be intense scrutiny of the safety profile, with particular attention to the risk of infections.

Not all new pathways turn out to be successful. Inhibition of the Spleen Tyrosine Kinase pathway (SyK) has also been investigated, however the results of the phase three trial revealed efficacy levels below that deemed necessary for the drug to move to market and so this pathway has fallen off the radar for RA [7].

PDE4 Inhibitors

Phosphodiesterase 4 (PDE4) is a member of the larger family of phosphodiesterases. PDE4 is an intracellular molecule that is involved in the hydrolysis of cyclic AMP within immune cells, enabling subsequent signaling pathway activation. Blocking PDE4 has the potential to suppress a wide range of inflammatory pathways including specific Th1 and Th2 responses. Inhibitors of the PDE pathways have been available for many years: theophylline is an example of a non-selective phosphodiesterase inhibitor. Such agents have been limited in use because of a very narrow therapeutic window and a high rate of adverse events. However, newer compounds that selectively target phosphodiesterase subfamilies are emerging as important anti-inflammatory agents.

Apremilast is a potent and selective PDE4 inhibitor that has already shown efficacy in PsA (with a US licence granted and a European license pending) and results of a large phase 3 trial in RA currently awaited.

Future Targets

The examples mentioned already represent pathways where a drug is already in a late stage of development. However there are numerous other drugs in various stages of development that will filter through in the coming years. In particular the relatively recent discovery of a new subset of T cells, the Th17 class, that appear to be specifically implicated in autoimmune disease is of great interest [8]. Two corresponding cytokines, IL-17 and IL-22 have been identified as circulating potential targets to inhibit the Th17 pathway. Several blocking agents are currently under study across a wide range of autoimmune diseases.

References

1. Dranitsaris G, Amir E, Dorward K. Biosimilars of biological drug therapies: regulatory, clinical and commercial considerations. Drugs. 2011;71:1527–36.
2. Scheinberg MA, Kay J. The advent of biosimilar therapies in rheumatology–"O brave new world". Nat Rev Rheumatol. 2012;8:430–6.
3. Schiestl M, Stangler T, Torella C, Cepeljnik T, Toll H, Grau R. Acceptable changes in quality attributes of glycosylated biopharmaceuticals. Nat Biotechnol. 2011;29:310–2.
4. Radstake TR, Svenson M, Eijsbouts AM, van den Hoogen FH, Enevold C, van Riel PL, et al. Formation of antibodies against infliximab and adalimumab strongly correlates with functional drug levels and clinical responses in rheumatoid arthritis. Ann Rheum Dis. 2009;68:1739–45.
5. Finckh A, Simard JF, Gabay C, Guerne PA, Physicians S. Evidence for differential acquired drug resistance to anti-tumour necrosis factor agents in rheumatoid arthritis. Ann Rheum Dis. 2006;65: 746–52.

6. Lee EB, Fleischmann R, Hall S, Wilkinson B, Bradley JD, Gruben D, et al. Tofacitinib versus methotrexate in rheumatoid arthritis. N Engl J Med. 2014;370:2377–86.

7. Weinblatt ME, Genovese MC, Ho M, Hollis S, Rosiak-Jedrychowicz K, Kavanaugh A, et al. Effects of fostamatinib, an oral spleen tyrosine kinase inhibitor, in rheumatoid arthritis patients with an inadequate response to methotrexate: results from a phase III, multicenter, randomized, double-blind, placebo-controlled, parallel-group study. Arthritis Rheumatol. 2014. doi:10.1002/art.38851.

8. Harrington LE, Hatton RD, Mangan PR, Turner H, Murphy TL, Murphy KM, et al. Interleukin 17-producing CD4+ effector T cells develop via a lineage distinct from the T helper type 1 and 2 lineages. Nat Immunol. 2005;6:1123–32. doi:10.1038/ni1254.

Chapter 14
Stratified Medicine in Inflammatory Arthritis

Abstract Stratified medicine involves identifying groups of patients that are likely to benefit from certain treatment strategies. As inflammatory arthritis patients vary greatly in their prognosis and which treatments they respond to, a stratified approach to their management is needed. A number of clinical and genetic factors have been identified that can be used to predict an inflammatory arthritis patient's likely prognosis and response to treatment. This chapter will provide an overview of these factors in patients with RA, PsA and AS. It will describe how current International guidelines recommend using these factors to make treatment intensity decisions in inflammatory arthritis patients.

Keywords Stratified Medicine • Prognostic • Biomarkers • ACPA • Genetics

What Is Stratified Medicine?

Stratified medicine involves the identification of patent subgroups that either have distinct mechanisms of disease or are likely to respond to particular treatments [1].

I.C. Scott et al., *Inflammatory Arthritis in Clinical Practice*,
DOI 10.1007/978-1-4471-6648-1_14,
© Springer-Verlag London 2015

This approach allows the identification of groups of patients that are most likely to benefit from specific management strategies. In short, it ensures that the right patient gets the right treatment at the right time [1], which is the holy grail of modern clinical practice.

Why Stratified Medicine Is Needed in Inflammatory Arthritis Patients

The inflammatory arthropathies are highly heterogeneous disorders. This heterogeneity can be considered from two perspectives:

1. *Variability in Disease Course*

    Inflammatory arthritis patients vary greatly in their disease course. Some patients have an aggressive condition, characterised by the early development of radiological damage and disability. Others have a much milder course with normal X-rays and no functional impairment.
2. *Variability in Treatment Responses*

    Inflammatory arthritis patients vary greatly in their treatment responses. One key example is that one third of RA patients will fail to achieve an ACR20 response after being treated with anti-TNF, which is the first line treatment in active disease not responding to DMARD therapy [2].

This clinical heterogeneity means that for inflammatory arthritis patients to receive high quality care a stratified approach to their management is needed, using clinical characteristics and biomarkers to identify groups of patients particularly likely to respond to specific therapeutic strategies. This stratified approach contrasts with current UK guidelines for inflammatory arthritis patients, which recommend empirical practice managing patients according to the same treatment pathway.

Existing Research in Stratified Medicine in Inflammatory Arthritis Patients

A substantial amount of research relevant to stratified medicine has been undertaken in RA patients. Numerous factors have been shown to associate with disease outcomes and treatment responses. A few research groups have attempted to combine these within prediction models that can be used to inform patient care. The evidence base for stratified medicine in other forms of inflammatory arthritis is more limited, although several factors have been shown to predict disease outcomes and treatment responses in PsA and AS patients. This chapter will therefore primarily focus on stratified medicine in RA. It will provide a brief overview of relevant prognostic factors in non-RA inflammatory arthropathies.

Predictors of Disease Course in RA

Serology

RF and ACPA are established predictors of RA severity. Their presence associates with a more severe disease course characterised by higher rates of radiological damage and extra-articular manifestations. In one observational study of 135 early RA patients, individuals with a persistently positive RF had greater X-ray damage, disease activity and disability and required more aggressive treatment [3]. Similarly in a cohort study of 93 early RA patients identified amongst blood donors, the presence of ACPA prior to and at disease onset associated with worse radiological outcomes [4].

Smoking

There is some evidence that smoking influences RA severity. In one study of 100 early RA patients observed over 24 months smokers had more swollen and tender joints, when compared to non-smokers [5]. The impact of smoking is, however, difficult to assess as it predispose to ACPA formation, which could mediate its effect on disease severity.

Alcohol

Two observational studies have indicated that alcohol consumption may reduce RA severity. In one study of 873 RA cases, more frequent alcohol intake significantly associated with lower DAS28-CRP, Larsen and HAQ scores [6]. In another large observational study of 2,908 RA patients a J-shaped dose-response effect was seen with occasional/daily drinkers having less X-ray progression compared with non-drinkers/heavy drinkers [7].

Social Deprivation

Several studies have observed a correlation between social deprivation and poor RA outcomes. In 869 patients from the Early Rheumatoid Arthritis Study (ERAS) higher social deprivation scores associated with higher HAQ scores and joint counts [8]. This effect may be driven by other lifestyle factors that associate with low socioeconomic status such as smoking.

Gender

RA may be more severe in women. In a prospective study of 225 women and 67 men with seropositive early RA, women had worse disease progression over 2 years with higher DAS28 scores despite receiving similar therapy to men; men had higher remission rates [9]. In another Swedish study women had significantly higher DAS28 and HAQ scores compared with males at all time-points over 5 years [10].

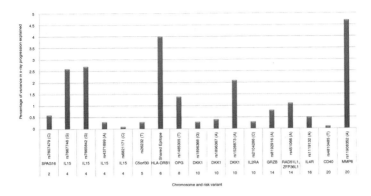

Figure 14.1 Validated genetic predictors of RA radiological progression- their association with 6-year changes in X-ray scores in 239 Dutch early RA patients. The risk allele for each SNP is given in the brackets; X-ray progression measured using the 6-year change in Sharp/van der Heidje scores; the variance of each variant is from a univariate analysis (Figure produced using data reported by Van Steenbergen et al. [11])

Genetics

A number of studies have tried to identify genetic markers that can be used to predict RA severity. Most have focussed on genetic associations with X-ray progression. To date 12 genetic loci that associate with radiological progression have been identified and replicated [11]. In a Dutch study of 426 early RA patients, these genetic variants explained approximately 18 % of the variance in X-ray progression, measured as the change in the Sharp-van der Heijde score over 6 years (Fig. 14.1). Most loci had minor effects on X-ray progression. Additionally, their impact was reduced when adjusting for traditional prognostic factors such as age, gender and ACPA, suggesting that their effects may be partially mediated by these clinical factors.

Predicting RA Severity

Several research groups have attempted to combine these predictive factors in "prediction models", which can be used to predict which patients are likely to have rapid radiological progression (RRP). One research group developed a model that included the predictors CRP, erosion score and serology (RF and ACPA). Their model was able to identify groups of patients at a very high or low risk of RRP. The highest risk group had a risk of RRP of 78 %; the lowest risk group had a risk of RRP of just 1 % [12]. Although this suggests stratifying RA patients to prognostic groups is possible, these prediction models have limited abilities to correctly discriminate radiological progressors from non-progressors. Additionally they have mainly been developed and tested in a single dataset and require validation in external cohorts.

Predictors of Treatment Responses in RA

Gender

Research suggests that males probably respond better to methotrexate than females. A systematic review of studies reporting predictors of methotrexate response found that women were up to three times less likely to have a good clinical response when treated with methotrexate compared to men [13].

Data from the British Society for Rheumatology Biologics Register (which collects clinical data on patients receiving biologic drugs in the UK) suggests that women may also respond less well to anti-TNF therapy. In this analysis of nearly 3,000 RA patients female gender associated with a reduced odds of remission with etanercept (OR 0.61; 95 % CI 0.38–0.94) and infliximab (OR 0.60; 95 % CI 0.40–0.89) treatment [14].

Smoking

Several studies have reported that smoking reduces the efficacy of methotrexate and anti-TNF treatment. One example is the Epidemiological Investigation of Rheumatoid Arthritis

(EIRA) study, undertaken in Sweden [15]. In this analysis current smokers were less likely to attain a good response when receiving both methotrexate and anti-TNF therapy. Interestingly, a history of previous smoking did not affect treatment responses.

Serology

Although RF and ACPA do not clearly affect responses to DMARD treatment there is good evidence that the requirement for intensive combination treatment differs between RA patients with and without ACPA. In an analysis of 431 patients with early, active RA enrolled to the Combination Anti-Rheumatic Drugs in Early RA (CARDERA) trial, only ACPA-positive patients benefited from intensive combination treatment [16]. No benefit beyond monotherapy with methotrexate was observed in ACPA-negative patients. This is demonstrated in Fig. 14.2, which shows mean changes from baseline in modified Larsen scores (measuring X-ray damage) in ACPA-positive and ACPA-negative patients receiving combination treatment or methotrexate monotherapy over 2-years. Combination treatment significantly reduced X-ray progression beyond methotrexate monotherapy at all time-points in ACPA-positive patients. By contrast ACPA-negative patients had minimal X-ray progression irrespective of the treatment strategy used.

There is some evidence that ACPA status can also predict which patients are most likely to respond to biologic drugs. Rituximab appears more effective in seropositive (RF and/or ACPA-positive) patients, with a meta-analysis of four RCTs demonstrating a significantly greater reduction in DAS28 scores between seropositive and seronegative RA patients at 24 weeks [17]. By contrast TNF-inhibitors seem more efficacious in ACPA-negative disease. In an analysis of the UK Biologics Registry, ACPA-negative patients had a 0.39 (95 % CI 0.07–0.71) greater mean improvement in DAS28 with anti-TNF compared with ACPA-positive patients [18].

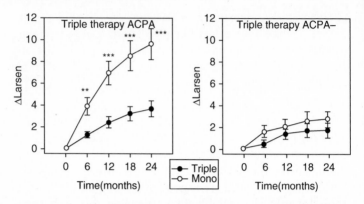

FIGURE 14.2 Impact of ACPA status on responses to combination treatment in 431 early active RA patients in the CARDERA trial. Δ*Larsen* mean change in Larsen scores from study baseline, *Triple* triple therapy with methotrexate, prednisolone and ciclosporin, *Mono* methotrexate monotherapy, standard error bars are shown; *indicates significance between treatment groups at $P < 0.05$; ** indicates significance between treatment groups at $P \leq 0.01$; *** indicates significance between treatment groups at $P \leq 0.001$ (Figure adapted with permission from Seegobin et al. (available at http://arthritis-research.com/content/16/1/R13) [16], licensed under the Creative Commons Attribution License; figure amended to include only final pair of graphs)

Overall the impact of ACPA status on biologic responses is modest, and is of too small an effect size to guide clinical decision making on its own.

Disease Duration

It is established that treating RA in its very early stages improves patient outcomes. This concept, known as the "window of opportunity", is demonstrated in a meta-analysis of 14 RCTs evaluating predictors of DMARD responses [19]. The percentages of patients attaining an ACR 20 response with active treatment comprised 53, 43, 44, 38 and 35 % for patients with disease durations of <1 year, 1–2 years, 2–5 years, 5–10 years and >10 years, respectively.

Genetics

Attempts to identify genetic predictors of methotrexate response have focussed on the methotrexate cellular pathway. Their results have been inconsistent and no clear genetic marker that predicts methotrexate responses has been identified [20]. One validated genetic marker that associates with anti-TNF response has been identified. In this study of nearly 3,000 RA patients one SNP (rs6427528) at the *1q23* locus associated with changes in DAS28 in patients receiving etanercept ($P = 8 \times 10^{-8}$) [21].

Prediction Models for Treatment Responses in RA

One research group has developed a model that predicts methotrexate responses in patients with early, active RA [22]. Eight predictive factors (four clinical and four genetic) were combined to generate a clinical score (ranging from 0 to 11.5) predicting the probability of a treatment response, defined as a DAS of ≤ 2.4 at 6 months. Using a score cut-off of ≤ 3.5 points for treatment responders provided a true positive rate of 95 %; using a score cut-off of ≥ 6 points for non-responders provided a true negative response rate of 86 %. The model had modest ability to discriminate between responders and non-responders, with an AUC value of 0.79. One major limitation of the model was that it classified approximately half of actual responders as having an "intermediate risk" of responding, which is not clinically useful. Further work is required to identify other risk factors for methotrexate response, which should reduce the size of the intermediate risk group. Similar prediction models are yet to be developed for other DMARDs or biologics.

Stratified Medicine in Non-RA Inflammatory Arthropathies

Psoriatic Arthritis

In PsA a number of clinical factors have been shown to predict an individual's disease course. Examples include:

1. Significant inflammation at first presentation- evidence of significant inflammation at a patient's first visit, for example high swollen joint counts, has been shown to associate with a more aggressive disease course [23]
2. Dactylitis- the presence of dactylitis, which is a common occurrence in PsA patients, appears to influence disease severity, as it correlates with greater radiological progression in the affected digit [24]
3. Smoking, an older age at diagnosis and female gender- these clinical factors have all been linked to higher levels of disability [25].

Genetic associations with PsA outcomes are limited to small studies of the HLA locus. In 276 PsA patients followed-up over 14-years the HLA antigens B27, B39, and DQw3 associated with disease progression [26]. In another study of 101 Italian PsA patients, DQw3 also associated with more severe disease [27]. Large studies with replication across multiple populations are required to validate the prognostic relevance of these findings.

Several studies have examined predictors of treatment responses in PsA patients. In one clinical trial of adalimumab therapy in active PsA patients, lower disability levels, male gender, an absence of steroid therapy and higher patient reported pain levels strongly associated with the attainment of an ACR50 and good EULAR response to treatment at 3 months [28]. An analysis of data from the Danish biologics registry identified baseline CRP levels as the dominant predictor of anti-TNF therapy response [29]. In this study, 1 in 7 patients with normal CRP levels at treatment initiation achieved an ACR70 response with anti-TNF. In contrast 1 in 3 patients whose CRP level was elevated at treatment initiation attained an ACR70 response.

Ankylosing Spondylitis

A number of clinical factors have been linked to the severity of radiological damage in AS patients. These include male gender, the presence of an inflammatory arthritis affecting the hip joint and a history of iritis, which have all been linked to more severe radiological damage in the spine.

A number of factors have also been linked to the severity of AS defined using Bath AS Disease Activity Index (BASDAI) and Bath AS Functional Index (BASFI) scores. In one study of 635 patients treated with anti-TNF, the variables age, BASFI scores, enthesitis, treatment, CRP and HLA-B27 genotype associated with BASDAI50 (50 % reduction in BASDAI scores) responses [30]. In another study of 311 AS patients, the variables smoking, BASDAI scores and the extent of radiological damage seen in the spine, hip and sacroiliac joints predicted BASFI scores in patients with established disease [31].

Current Use of Stratified Medicine in Inflammatory Arthritis Patients

Current UK clinical guidelines from the National Institute for Health and Care Excellence (NICE) recommend treating all inflammatory arthritis patients according to a single treatment pathway. By contrast International guidelines from the American College of Rheumatology (ACR) and European League Against Rheumatism (EULAR) advocate using a stratified approach to treatment decisions in inflammatory arthritis patients, reserving aggressive treatment for patients with adverse prognostic features. Two examples of this stratified approach are as follows.

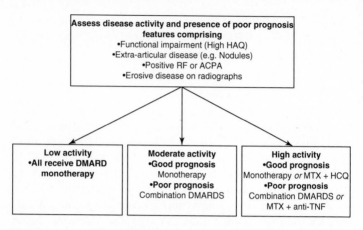

FIGURE 14.3 ACR guidelines for the management of early RA patients advocating a stratified approach based on poor prognosis features. *HAQ* health assessment questionnaire, *RF* rheumatoid factor, *ACPA* antibodies to citrullinated protein antigens, *DMARD* disease-modifying anti-rheumatic drug, *MTX* methotrexate, *HCQ* hydroxychloroquine, *TNF* tumour necrosis factor (Figure based on 2012 ACR guidelines [32])

1. *2012 ACR guidelines for early RA treatment*

    Current American guidelines for the management of RA patients within the first 6 months of their disease recommend basing treatment intensity decisions on a patient's disease activity and the presence or absence of poor prognostic features (Fig. 14.3) [32].

2. *2012 EULAR guidelines for psoriatic arthritis patient management*

    Recent EULAR guidelines advocate NSAIDs as a first line therapy in most PsA patients, with DMARDs initiated in non-responders. However, they also recommend that in those patients with active disease (defined as ≥1 tender and inflamed joint) and poor prognostic markers, DMARDs should be instituted as a first line therapy [33]. Suggested poor prognostic factors comprise ≥5 active joints, elevated acute phase reactants, progressive radiographic damage, previous steroid use, loss of function and diminished quality of life.

Conclusion

Stratified medicine is an area of emerging importance in the management of inflammatory arthritis patients. Many poor prognostic factors have been identified, particularly in RA patients, which can be used to identify patients requiring more aggressive treatment. This knowledge is reflected in current International guidelines for managing RA and PsA patients, which advocate reserving intensive treatment for poor prognosis patients with active disease. By contrast knowledge of which factors predict responses to specific medications is more limited. Further research is required to better define relevant predictive factors in inflammatory arthritis patients and to develop and validate prediction models that combine these factors to identify patient groups likely to respond to certain therapies.

References

1. Medical Research Council. MRC website. 2014. [Internet] Available at: http://www.mrc.ac.uk/Ourresearch/ResearchInitiatives/StratifiedMedicine/index.htm. Accessed 19 Apr 2014.
2. Rubbert-Roth A, Finckh A. Treatment options in patients with rheumatoid arthritis failing initial TNF inhibitor therapy: a critical review. Arthritis Res Ther. 2009;11 Suppl 1:S1.
3. van Zeben D, Hazes JM, Zwinderman AH, Cats A, van der Voort EA, Breedveld FC. Clinical significance of rheumatoid factors in early rheumatoid arthritis: results of a follow up study. Ann Rheum Dis. 1992;51:1029–35.
4. Berglin E, Johansson T, Sundin U, Jidell E, Wadell G, Hallmans G, et al. Radiological outcome in rheumatoid arthritis is predicted by presence of antibodies against cyclic citrullinated peptide before and at disease onset, and by IgA-RF at disease onset. Ann Rheum Dis. 2006;65:453–8.
5. Manfredsdottir VF, Vikingsdottir T, Jonsson T, Geirsson AJ, Kjartansson O, Heimisdottir M, et al. The effects of tobacco smoking and rheumatoid factor seropositivity on disease activity and joint damage in early rheumatoid arthritis. Rheumatology (Oxford). 2006;45:734–40.

6. Maxwell JR, Gowers IR, Moore DJ, Wilson AG. Alcohol consumption is inversely associated with risk and severity of rheumatoid arthritis. Rheumatology (Oxford). 2010;49:2140–6.
7. Nissen MJ, Gabay C, Scherer A, Finckh A, Swiss Clinical Quality Management Project in Rheumatoid A. The effect of alcohol on radiographic progression in rheumatoid arthritis. Arthritis Rheum. 2010;62:1265–72.
8. ERAS Study Group. Socioeconomic deprivation and rheumatoid disease: what lessons for the health service? ERAS Study Group. Early Rheumatoid Arthritis Study. Ann Rheum Dis. 2000;59:794–9.
9. Jawaheer D, Maranian P, Park G, Lahiff M, Amjadi SS, Paulus HE. Disease progression and treatment responses in a prospective DMARD-naive seropositive early rheumatoid arthritis cohort: does gender matter? J Rheumatol. 2010;37:2475–85.
10. Ahlmen M, Svensson B, Albertsson K, Forslind K, Hafstrom I, Barfot Study Group. Influence of gender on assessments of disease activity and function in early rheumatoid arthritis in relation to radiographic joint damage. Ann Rheum Dis. 2010;69:230–3.
11. van Steenbergen HW, Tsonaka R, Huizinga TW, le Cessie S, van der Helm-van Mil AM. Predicting the severity of joint damage in rheumatoid arthritis; the contribution of genetic factors. Ann Rheum Dis. 2014. [Epub Ahead of Print].
12. Visser K, Goekoop-Ruiterman YPM, de Vries-Bouwstra JK, Ronday HK, Seys PEH, Kerstens PJSM, et al. A matrix risk model for the prediction of rapid radiographic progression in patients with rheumatoid arthritis receiving different dynamic treatment strategies: post hoc analyses from the BeSt study. Ann Rheum Dis. 2010;69:1333–7.
13. Drouin J, Haraoui B, e Initiative Group. Predictors of clinical response and radiographic progression in patients with rheumatoid arthritis treated with methotrexate monotherapy. J Rheumatol. 2010;37:1405–10.
14. Hyrich KL, Watson KD, Silman AJ, Symmons DP, British Society for Rheumatology Biologics Register. Predictors of response to anti-TNF-alpha therapy among patients with rheumatoid arthritis: results from the British Society for Rheumatology Biologics Register. Rheumatology (Oxford). 2006;45:1558–65.
15. Saevarsdottir S, Wedren S, Seddighzadeh M, Bengtsson C, Wesley A, Lindblad S, et al. Patients with early rheumatoid arthritis who smoke are less likely to respond to treatment with

methotrexate and tumor necrosis factor inhibitors: observations from the Epidemiological Investigation of Rheumatoid Arthritis and the Swedish Rheumatology Register cohorts. Arthritis Rheum. 2011;63:26–36.

16. Seegobin SD, Ma MH, Dahanayake C, Cope AP, Scott DL, Lewis CM, et al. ACPA-positive and ACPA-negative rheumatoid arthritis differ in their requirements for combination DMARDs and corticosteroids: secondary analysis of a randomized controlled trial. Arthritis Res Ther. 2014;16:R13.

17. Isaacs JD, Cohen SB, Emery P, Tak PP, Wang J, Lei G, et al. Effect of baseline rheumatoid factor and anticitrullinated peptide antibody serotype on rituximab clinical response: a meta-analysis. Ann Rheum Dis. 2013;72:329–36.

18. Potter C, Hyrich KL, Tracey A, Lunt M, Plant D, Symmons DPM, et al. Association of rheumatoid factor and anti-cyclic citrullinated peptide positivity, but not carriage of shared epitope or PTPN22 susceptibility variants, with anti-tumour necrosis factor response in rheumatoid arthritis. Ann Rheum Dis. 2009;68: 69–74.

19. Anderson JJ, Wells G, Verhoeven AC, Felson DT. Factors predicting response to treatment in rheumatoid arthritis: the importance of disease duration. Arthritis Rheum. 2000;43:22–9.

20. Malik F, Ranganathan P. Methotrexate pharmacogenetics in rheumatoid arthritis: a status report. Pharmacogenomics. 2013;14:305–14.

21. Cui J, Stahl EA, Saevarsdottir S, Miceli C, Diogo D, Trynka G, et al. Genome-wide association study and gene expression analysis identifies CD84 as a predictor of response to etanercept therapy in rheumatoid arthritis. PLoS Genet. 2013;9: e1003394.

22. Wessels JA, van der Kooij SM, le Cessie S, Kievit W, Barerra P, Allaart CF, et al. A clinical pharmacogenetic model to predict the efficacy of methotrexate monotherapy in recent-onset rheumatoid arthritis. Arthritis Rheum. 2007;56:1765–75.

23. Gladman DD, Farewell VT, Nadeau C. Clinical indicators of progression in psoriatic arthritis: multivariate relative risk model. J Rheumatol. 1995;22:675–9.

24. Brockbank JE, Stein M, Schentag CT, Gladman DD. Dactylitis in psoriatic arthritis: a marker for disease severity? Ann Rheum Dis. 2005;64:188–90.

25. Tillett W, Jadon D, Shaddick G, Cavill C, Korendowych E, de Vries CS, et al. Smoking and delay to diagnosis are associated

with poorer functional outcome in psoriatic arthritis. Ann Rheum Dis. 2013;72:1358–61.

26. Gladman DD, Farewell VT. The role of HLA antigens as indicators of disease progression in psoriatic arthritis. Multivariate relative risk model. Arthritis Rheum. 1995;38:845–50.

27. Salvarani C, Macchioni PL, Zizzi F, Mantovani W, Rossi F, Baricchi R, et al. Clinical subgroups and HLA antigens in Italian patients with psoriatic arthritis. Clin Exp Rheumatol. 1989;7:391–6.

28. Van den Bosch F, Manger B, Goupille P, McHugh N, Rodevand E, Holck P, et al. Effectiveness of adalimumab in treating patients with active psoriatic arthritis and predictors of good clinical responses for arthritis, skin and nail lesions. Ann Rheum Dis. 2010;69:394–9.

29. Glintborg B, Ostergaard M, Dreyer L, Krogh NS, Tarp U, Hansen MS, et al. Treatment response, drug survival, and predictors thereof in 764 patients with psoriatic arthritis treated with anti-tumor necrosis factor alpha therapy: results from the nationwide Danish DANBIO registry. Arthritis Rheum. 2011;63:382–90.

30. Vastesaeger N, van der Heijde D, Inman RD, Wang Y, Deodhar A, Hsu B, et al. Predicting the outcome of ankylosing spondylitis therapy [Erratum appears in Ann Rheum Dis. 2012 Aug;71(8):1434]. Ann Rheum Dis. 2011;70:973–81.

31. Doran MF, Brophy S, MacKay K, Taylor G, Calin A. Predictors of longterm outcome in ankylosing spondylitis. J Rheumatol. 2003;30:316–20.

32. Singh JA, Furst DE, Bharat A, Curtis JR, Kavanaugh AF, Kremer JM, et al. 2012 update of the 2008 American College of Rheumatology recommendations for the use of disease-modifying antirheumatic drugs and biologic agents in the treatment of rheumatoid arthritis. Arthritis Care Res. 2012;64:625–39.

33. Gossec L, Smolen JS, Gaujoux-Viala C, Ash Z, Marzo-Ortega H, van der Heijde D, et al. European League Against Rheumatism recommendations for the management of psoriatic arthritis with pharmacological therapies. Ann Rheum Dis. 2012;71:4–12.

Index

I.C. Scott et al., *Inflammatory Arthritis in Clinical Practice*,   207
DOI 10.1007/978-1-4471-6648-1,
© Springer-Verlag London 2015

Printed by Printforce, the Netherlands